CORTISOL DETOX MEAL PLAN

28 Days Meal Plan and 100+ Easy, Delicious Recipes to Help Restore Hormonal Balance, Reduce Stress, Lose Weight, and Improve Your Health

Keyla Leach

Copyright© 2024 by Keyla Leach

All rights reserved worldwide.

No part of this book may be reproduced or transmitted in any form or by any means, electronic or mechanical, including photo- copying, recording or by any information storage and retrieval system, without written permission from the publisher, except for the inclusion of brief quotations in a review.

Warning-Disclaimer

The purpose of this book is to educate and entertain. The author or publisher does not guarantee that anyone following the techniques, suggestions, tips, ideas, or strategies will become successful. The author and publisher shall have either liability or responsibility to anyone with respect to any loss or damage caused, or alleged to be caused, directly or indirectly by the information contained in this book.

Table of Contents

Stress is often our constant companion in the fast-paced world of today. Our bodies are under continuous stress from waking up to a buzzing alarm, navigating traffic, and juggling the demands of job, family, and personal objectives. While a certain amount of stress is normal, chronic stress negatively impacts our health, mostly via the hormone cortisol, which you may be familiar with. Cortisol, also called the "stress hormone," is an essential ingredient of our body's reaction to stress. Long-term increased cortisol levels, however, may cause several health problems, ranging from mood changes and weakened immunity to weight gain and exhaustion.

Welcome to the Cortisol Detox Diet Cookbook, a manual on using food to nurture your body and calm your mind. This book explores the connection between our eating habits and emotions, not diets. It all comes down to choosing foods to help your body cope with stress, maintain emotional stability, and replenish energy. This cookbook offers a route to holistic well-being by emphasizing cortisol-conscious meals and ingredients.

Understanding Cortisol and Its Role in Our Bodies

Cortisol is created by the adrenal glands, located above our kidneys, and released into the bloodstream during moments of stress. It is the body's natural reaction to what is known as the "fight-or-flight" scenario, supplying us with energy, increasing our alertness, and assisting us in dealing with immediate obstacles. However, when our bodies experience persistent stress, whether from job constraints, a lack of sleep, a bad diet, or mental strain, cortisol production may go into overdrive, overwhelming our system with this potent hormone.

An imbalance in cortisol levels may cause a range of health issues. These include weight gain, particularly around the midsection; exhaustion; a decreased immunological system; digestive problems; increased desires, particularly for high-sugar and high-fat meals; and even changes to our sleep patterns. Chronic stress and high cortisol levels may have a long-term impact on our mental health, making us feel more nervous, irritated, or even sad.

The foods we consume may greatly influence how our bodies regulate cortisol levels. We may improve our health by consuming foods and ingredients that help manage cortisol levels. This cookbook's recipes and nutritional suggestions have been meticulously created to give meals high in nutrients, low in processed sugars, balanced in healthy fats, and filled with vitamins, minerals, and antioxidants. These foods foster a healthy stress response and help you achieve a calmer, more balanced lifestyle.

The Science behind a Cortisol Detox Diet

The concept of a "detox" is frequently related to removing toxins from the body. In the case of a Cortisol Detox Diet, our primary goal is to reduce the stressors that can cause elevated cortisol levels. This entails selecting foods that work together with your body to maintain stable blood sugar levels, minimize inflammation, and promote adrenal health. Selecting meals high in fiber, antioxidants, omega-3 fatty acids, and key vitamins gives your body the skills to deal with daily pressures.

Blood sugar equilibrium is a fundamental theme of the Cortisol Detox Diet. When blood sugar levels vary dramatically due to ingesting high-sugar or highly processed foods, cortisol is called upon to assist in stabilizing them, which can result in an unwanted surge in cortisol levels. On the other hand, meals high in complex carbs, lean proteins, and healthy fats aid in maintaining blood sugar levels and reduce needless cortisol release. Furthermore, antioxidants found in fruits, vegetables, and whole grains help battle oxidative stress, damaging cells and increasing cortisol levels. The recipes in this book are designed to reduce these stressors, allowing your body to "detox" from the frequent cortisol spikes.

How to Manage Cortisol Based on Science

Cortisol management needs lifestyle changes, nutritional decisions, and mindfulness activities. Understanding the elements that regulate cortisol allows us to make daily decisions that promote a calmer, healthier body and mind. Here's a closer look at the science behind cortisol management and practical strategies you may take to regulate this stress hormone.

1. Prioritize Balanced Nutrition

Nutrition is an essential ingredient of cortisol regulation. What we consume can either balance or increase cortisol levels. Certain nutrients are renowned for their potential to regulate blood sugar, reduce inflammation, and promote adrenal health—all of which contribute to cortisol management.

- ✓ **Complex Carbohydrates:** Whole grains, lentils, and root vegetables give a continuous energy supply, avoiding blood sugar spikes and crashes that might cause cortisol release. According to studies, meals high in complex carbohydrates can lower cortisol and induce calm by stabilizing blood glucose levels.
- ✓ **Healthy Fats:** Omega-3 fatty acids, found in salmon, walnuts, chia seeds, and flaxseeds, are believed to have anti-inflammatory properties. Because inflammation can raise cortisol levels, omega-3s help combat inflammation and support a healthy stress response.

- ✓ **Magnesium-rich foods:** Magnesium is an essential mineral that regulates over 300 enzymatic activities, including cortisol levels. Magnesium-rich foods, such as leafy greens, nuts, seeds, and avocados, aid in relaxing the nervous system and reducing cortisol secretion under stressful conditions.
- ✓ **Vitamin C:** According to research, vitamin C-rich foods such as bell peppers, citrus fruits, and strawberries can help lower cortisol levels, particularly during physical or psychological stress. Vitamin C also promotes adrenal health, which is necessary for proper cortisol production.
- ✓ **Adaptogenic Herbs:** Adaptogens are plants that assist the body in adapting to stress. Examples include ashwagandha, rhodiola, and holy basil. According to research, these herbs can help to normalize cortisol levels by supporting adrenal function and increasing stress resilience.

2. Keep a regular eating schedule

Regular meal scheduling is equally crucial as food selection. Irregular eating patterns can cause variations in blood sugar levels, elevating cortisol. According to research, skipping meals might cause a drop in blood sugar, increasing the release of cortisol to compensate. To maintain blood sugar stability, eat at predictable times throughout the day and incorporate protein, healthy fats, and fiber in each meal. This technique lowers the likelihood of cortisol surges and provides a consistent energy source throughout the day.

3. Prioritize quality sleep

Sleep is one of the most effective ways to regulate cortisol levels. Cortisol levels naturally decline during deep sleep, allowing the body to rest and recover. However, poor sleep interrupts the regular cycle, keeping cortisol levels high. Chronic sleep loss can cause higher cortisol levels over time, making stress management more difficult.

According to studies, humans require approximately 7-9 hours of sleep per night for healthy cortisol regulation. Good sleep hygiene, such as sticking to a consistent sleep schedule, limiting screen time before bed, and providing a relaxing resting environment, can enhance sleep quality and, as a result, manage cortisol.

4. Exercise mindfully

Physical activity is a well-known stress reliever that, when used in moderation, is beneficial for cortisol management. Exercise produces endorphins, which can counteract cortisol and relieve stress. However, intense or sustained activity might cause a temporary spike in cortisol levels.

The idea is to engage in enjoyable activities while listening to your body's requirements. Low-to-moderate intensity exercises, including walking, swimming, yoga, and Pilates, have been demonstrated to reduce cortisol levels and increase mood. High-intensity exercise can be beneficial but should be done in short, regulated bursts to avoid chronic cortisol surges.

5. Practice Mindful Relaxation Techniques

Mindful relaxation techniques such as meditation, deep breathing, and mindfulness practices significantly impact cortisol. According to research, even a few minutes of mindfulness meditation can reduce cortisol levels and boost activity in brain regions associated with calm and relaxation.

Breathing exercises, in particular, are simple to include in regular routines. Simple strategies, such as deep belly breathing, promote the parasympathetic nerve system, or "rest and digest" response, which can counteract the effects of stress and lower cortisol. Set aside 5-10 minutes daily for mindful relaxation to reap the most advantages.

6. Foster positive social connections

Positive social interactions and supportive connections have a major impact on cortisol levels. When we engage in meaningful relationships or spend time with loved ones, our bodies release oxytocin, sometimes known as the "bonding hormone." Oxytocin reduces cortisol levels and promotes calm.

Conversely, social isolation or damaged relationships can increase stress and cortisol levels. Making time for friends, family, or supportive community groups can help you maintain a good emotional balance and reduce stress.

7. Establish boundaries to manage external stressors

Work deadlines, financial constraints, social media, and continual contact contribute to modern life's potential stressors. If not managed well, these stressors can cause chronic cortisol increase. Setting boundaries for work, technology, and personal time can reduce stress.

Set clear periods for work, rest, and pleasure, and restrict screen use, particularly before bedtime. Creating designated "stress-free" moments where you disengage and engage in soothing activities might help reset cortisol levels and act as a stress buffer.

8. Stay hydrated

Dehydration is a lesser-known cause of cortisol release. When the body feels dehydrated, it enters a state of stress, resulting in a rise in cortisol. According to studies, even slight dehydration can cause cortisol to rise; therefore, staying hydrated is essential for stress management.

The Benefits of the Cortisol Detox Diet

The Cortisol Detox Diet is more than simply stress management; it is a comprehensive approach to wellness that promotes physical and mental equilibrium. This diet provides various benefits in addition to stress reduction by focusing on foods that control cortisol, stabilize blood sugar, reduce inflammation, and promote general adrenal health. Here are some of the main advantages of following the Cortisol Detox Diet.

1. Increased energy and less fatigue

One of the main advantages of the Cortisol Detox Diet is the possibility of enhanced energy and decreased weariness. Chronic stress and high cortisol levels can leave us feeling exhausted, both physically and emotionally. The foods in this diet help balance blood sugar, preventing energy crashes and keeping you steady throughout the day. Nutrient-dense foods, high in complex carbohydrates, healthy fats, and protein, provide long-term energy without the highs and lows associated with sugary or overly processed foods. The diet supports adrenal health, balances cortisol, and promotes a more constant, long-lasting energy flow.

2. Improved mood and emotional balance

High cortisol levels can cause anxiety, irritability, and even depression over time. The Cortisol Detox Diet promotes mood-regulating nutrients, including magnesium, tryptophan, and vitamin B. This diet can help decrease emotional swings caused by stress and cortisol imbalances by including these mood-enhancing foods. Additionally, lowering inflammation with anti-inflammatory foods can benefit brain health by boosting mental clarity and emotional stability. Many people report that when their nutrition improves, so does their sense of serenity and overall mood.

3. Weight Management and Reduced Belly Fat

Chronic stress and elevated cortisol levels are closely associated with weight gain, particularly in the abdomen. Cortisol raises hunger, particularly for comfort foods heavy in sugar and fat, resulting in weight gain. The Cortisol Detox Diet addresses this issue by prioritizing balanced meals that maintain steady blood sugar levels, lowering the chance of cortisol-induced cravings. This diet promotes healthy metabolism and simplifies managing or losing weight by focusing on satisfying, nutritious foods low in refined sugars.

Reducing belly fat is about more than just appearance; excess abdominal fat has been linked to an increased risk of heart disease, diabetes, and other health issues. The diet helps decrease these dangers by regulating cortisol levels and promoting physical and mental wellness.

4. Enhanced Immunity

The rise of chronic cortisol can impair the immune system, making us more prone to sickness. Over time, high cortisol levels might compromise immune function by diverting energy away from the immune response to prepare for anticipated threats. The Cortisol Detox Diet contains antioxidant-rich foods such as berries, leafy greens, and almonds, which boost the immune system and protect cells from damage. Vitamin C and zinc, which may be found in citrus fruits and pumpkin seeds, also promote immunological function and help the body fight infections more effectively. With stronger immunity, you'll be better able to stay healthy and resilient even when life's challenges emerge.

6. Reduced inflammation

Chronic inflammation can cause high cortisol levels, exacerbating stress and health difficulties. The Cortisol Detox Diet focuses on anti-inflammatory foods such as omega-3-rich fish, flaxseeds, and colorful fruits and vegetables, which assist in lowering systemic inflammation. The diet reduces inflammation, which helps prevent various health concerns such as cardiovascular disease, joint discomfort, and skin diseases. A diet low in inflammatory foods promotes mental clarity and can help alleviate the "brain fog" commonly associated with prolonged stress and inflammation.

7. Improved digestive health

Stress and high cortisol levels can disturb the digestive system, resulting in symptoms such as bloating, constipation, or even irritable bowel syndrome. High cortisol levels limit blood flow to the digestive organs, which impairs digestion and nutrient absorption. The Cortisol Detox Diet includes fiber-rich foods that maintain a healthy microbiota and improve digestion. Whole grains, leafy greens, and fermented foods (such as yogurt and kimchi) all include good bacteria and fibers that help with digestive function, reduce bloating, and improve regularity. Improved digestion also increases nutrient absorption, critical for general health and energy.

8. Improved Mental Focus and Cognitive Health

Cortisol is more than just a physical stress hormone; it also influences cognitive performance. Chronic stress and high cortisol levels can impair memory, diminish focus, and cause mental tiredness. The Cortisol Detox Diet contains brain-boosting nutrients such as omega-3 fatty acids, antioxidants, and B vitamins, which improve cognitive function and mental clarity. Omega-3s, for example, have been demonstrated to lower cortisol levels and boost brain function, while antioxidants shield brain cells from oxidative stress. Many people report that a diet rich in these nutrients improves their focus and mental resiliency.

9. Increased Resistance to Stress

One of the most significant advantages of the Cortisol Detox Diet is its ability to build resilience to stress over time. Building a foundation of balanced nutrition, stable blood sugar, and a good connection with food prepares your body to handle stress without raising cortisol levels. Furthermore, adaptogenic herbs such as ashwagandha and rhodiola help boost the body's resilience by promoting adrenal function and regulating cortisol levels. With a stronger body and mind, everyday pressures become easier to manage, and long-term stress has a lower impact on your well-being.

10. Long-term health benefits

High cortisol levels over time can contribute to a variety of chronic health issues, including heart disease, hypertension, type 2 diabetes, and mental disorders. Following the Cortisol Detox Diet, you manage stress and take preventative measures to avoid these long-term health problems. Each nutrient-dense meal contributes to the body's foundation, establishing a stronger immune system, lowering the risk of metabolic illnesses, and improving overall longevity. In this way, the Cortisol Detox Diet is a preventive health measure, allowing you to remain young and healthy for years.

Stress-Busting Overnight Oats

Prep Time: 10 minutes

Cook Time: Overnight chilling

Servings: 2

Ingredients

- 1 cup of rolled oats
- 1 cup of unsweetened almond milk
- 1 tbsp chia seeds
- 1/2 tsp cinnamon
- 1 tbsp honey or maple syrup (optional)
- 1/2 cup of mixed berries (fresh or frozen)
- 1/4 cup of chopped nuts
- 1 tbsp flaxseeds

Instructions

1. Mix the rolled oats, almond milk, chia seeds, and cinnamon in a medium bowl. Stir well to combine all of the ingredients.
2. Sweeten the mixture with honey or maple syrup, if desired.
3. Gently fold in the mixed berries and divide into two or airtight jars.
4. Seal the jars and chill overnight to let the oats soak and the flavors mingle.
5. In the morning, mix the oats thoroughly. Add more almond milk to correct the consistency if the mixture appears too thick.
6. Top each serving with chopped nuts and flaxseed.

Nutrition Information (per serving):

Calories: 350 Protein: 10 g Fat: 15 g Carbohydrates: 45 g Fiber: 9 g Sugar: 10 g

Anti-Inflammatory Turmeric Scramble

Prep Time: 5 minutes

Cook Time: 10 minutes

Servings: 2

Ingredients

- 4 large eggs
- 1/4 cup of milk
- 1 tsp turmeric powder
- 1/2 tsp black pepper
- 1/2 tsp salt
- 1 tbsp olive oil
- 1 small onion, finely chopped
- 1 clove garlic, minced
- 1/2 cup of chopped spinach
- 1/4 cup of chopped red bell pepper

Instructions

1. Combine the eggs, milk, turmeric, black pepper, and salt in a mixing bowl until well blended.
2. In a nonstick skillet, heat olive oil over medium heat.
3. Sauté the onion and garlic in the skillet until the onion is transparent, about 3 minutes.
4. Cook for 2 minutes, stirring in the chopped spinach and red bell pepper until wilted.
5. Pour the egg mixture into the skillet and let it sit for about a minute before gently stirring with a spatula to scramble the eggs until softly set and somewhat runny in parts.
6. When the eggs are done to your taste, remove them from the heat; residual heat will cause them to cook slightly longer.

Nutrition Information (per serving):

Calories: 250 Protein: 14 g Fat: 18 g Carbohydrates: 8 g Fiber: 2 g Sugar: 3 g

Blueberry Chia Pudding Delight

Prep Time: 10 minutes

Chill Time: 4 hours or overnight

Servings: 2

Ingredients

- 1/4 cup of chia seeds
- 1 cup of unsweetened almond milk
- 1/2 tsp vanilla extract
- 1 tbsp maple syrup or honey
- 1/2 cup of blueberries
- 1 tbsp shredded coconut (optional)

Instructions

1. Combine chia seeds, almond milk, and vanilla extract in a bowl. Stir well to incorporate and avoid clumps.
2. If desired, use maple syrup or honey to sweeten the mixture. Gently fold in the blueberries, dividing them equally.
3. Divide the mixture across two serving bowl or jars. Cover and chill for at least 4 hours, or overnight, until the pudding is thick and the chia seeds have absorbed the liquid.
4. Before serving, mix the pudding to achieve a uniform texture and top with shredded coconut for extra flavor and crunch.

Nutrition Information (per serving):

Calories: 200 Protein: 5 g Fat: 12 g Carbohydrates: 20 g Fiber: 8 g Sugar: 8 g

Avocado and Veggie Power Toast

Prep Time: 10 minutes

Cook Time: 5 minutes

Servings: 2

Ingredients

- 2 slices of whole-grain bread
- 1 ripe avocado
- 1/2 lemon, juiced
- Salt and pepper, to taste
- 1/2 cup of arugula
- 1/2 small cucumber, thinly sliced
- 4 cherry tomatoes, halved
- 1/4 red onion, thinly sliced
- 1 tbsp olive oil
- 1 tsp sesame seeds (optional)

Instructions

1. Toast the bread pieces till the desired doneness.
2. Combine the avocado, lemon juice, salt, and pepper in a small mixing bowl. Mash until smooth and spreadable.
3. Spread the mashed avocado equally over the toasted bread pieces. Place the arugula, cucumber slices, cherry tomato halves, and red onion slices on top of the avocado.
4. Drizzle olive oil over each slice of bread and sprinkle with sesame seeds, if desired.

Nutrition Information (per serving):

Calories: 320 Protein: 6 g Fat: 20 g Carbohydrates: 32 g Fiber: 10 g Sugar: 5 g

Almond Butter Banana Smoothie Bowl

Prep Time: 5 minutes

Servings: 2

Ingredients

- 2 ripe bananas, sliced and frozen
- 2 tbsp almond butter
- 1 cup of unsweetened almond milk
- 1/2 tsp vanilla extract
- 1 tbsp flaxseed meal
- Toppings:
- 1/4 cup of sliced almonds
- 1/4 cup of granola
- 1/2 banana, thinly sliced
- 1 tbsp chia seeds

Instructions

1. Blend the frozen banana slices, almond butter, almond milk, vanilla extract, and flaxseed meal. Blend until smooth and creamy.
2. Pour the smoothie into two bowls.
3. Top the smoothie bowls with sliced almonds, granola, banana slices, and chia seeds to add texture and taste.

Nutrition Information (per serving):

Calories: 400 Protein: 10 g Fat: 20 g Carbohydrates: 50 g Fiber: 12 g Sugar: 20 g

Coconut Quinoa Breakfast Porridge

Prep Time: 5 minutes

Cook Time: 15 minutes

Servings: 2

Ingredients

- 1/2 cup of quinoa, rinsed
- 1 cup of coconut milk
- 1/2 cup of water
- 1/4 tsp salt
- 1/2 tsp cinnamon
- 2 tbsp shredded coconut
- 1 tbsp honey or maple syrup (optional)
- Toppings:
- 1/4 cup of sliced bananas
- 1/4 cup of chopped nuts (almonds or pecans)
- Additional shredded coconut for garnish

Instructions

1. Mix the quinoa, coconut milk, water, and salt in a medium saucepan. Bring to a boil over medium-high heat.
2. Reduce the heat to low, cover, and cook for approximately 15 minutes until the quinoa is fully cooked and most of the liquid has been absorbed.
3. Remove from heat and add the cinnamon and shredded coconut. Sweeten with honey or maple syrup if preferred.
4. Divide the porridge into two bowls. Top with sliced bananas, chopped almonds, and more shredded coconut.

Nutrition Information (per serving):

Calories: 350 Protein: 8 g Fat: 18 g Carbohydrates: 40 g Fiber: 5 g Sugar: 10 g

Mushroom Spinach Frittata

Prep Time: 10 minutes

Cook Time: 20 minutes

Servings: 4

Ingredients

- 6 large eggs
- 1/4 cup of milk (dairy or plant-based)
- 1/2 tsp salt
- 1/4 tsp black pepper
- 1 tbsp olive oil
- 1 cup of fresh mushrooms, sliced
- 2 cups of spinach, washed and roughly chopped
- 1/2 onion, finely chopped
- 1 clove garlic, minced
- 1/2 cup of grated cheese

Instructions

1. Preheat the oven to 375° Fahrenheit (190° Celsius).
2. Combine eggs, milk, salt, and pepper in a large mixing bowl.
3. Heat the olive oil in a 10-inch oven-safe skillet over medium heat. Sauté the onions and garlic until they are transparent, approximately 3 minutes.
4. Cook until the mushrooms soften and release their juices, approximately 5 minutes. Add the spinach and simmer for approximately 2 minutes or until wilted.
5. Pour the egg mixture over the veggies in the skillet. Sprinkle with cheese if using.
6. Cook without stirring for 3 minutes or until the edges begin to firm.
7. Place the pan in the oven for 12-15 minutes or until the frittata is set and faintly browned on top.

Nutrition Information (per serving):

Calories: 220 Protein: 14 g Fat: 15 g Carbohydrates: 5 g Fiber: 1 g Sugar: 2 g

Chia Seed Pancakes with Berries

Prep Time: 10 minutes

Cook Time: 15 minutes

Servings: 4

Ingredients

- 1 cup of whole wheat flour
- 2 tbsp chia seeds
- 1 tbsp baking powder
- 1/2 tsp salt
- 1 cup of almond milk (or milk of choice)
- 1 large egg
- 1 tbsp maple syrup or honey
- 1 tsp vanilla extract
- 1 cup of mixed berries (blueberries, strawberries, or raspberries)
- 1 tbsp coconut oil or butter for cooking

Instructions

1. Combine the flour, chia seeds, baking powder, and salt in a large bowl.
2. Mix the almond milk, egg, maple syrup, and vanilla extract in a separate bowl until completely blended.
3. Pour the wet ingredients into the dry ingredients and mix until barely mixed. Fold in half of the berries, reserving the remainder for topping.
4. Heat a nonstick pan or griddle over medium heat, then add coconut oil or butter.
5. Pour 1/4 cup of batter into the skillet for each pancake. Cook for 2-3 minutes until bubbles appear on the surface. Flip and heat for 2 minutes or until golden brown and well done.
6. Repeat with the remaining batter, using more oil or butter as required.
7. Top the pancakes with the remaining berries and sprinkle with maple syrup or honey if preferred.

Nutrition Information (per serving):

Calories: 250 Protein: 7 g Fat: 8 g Carbohydrates: 35 g Fiber: 6 g Sugar: 8 g

Sweet Potato and Kale Hash

Prep Time: 10 minutes

Cook Time: 20 minutes

Servings: 2

Ingredients

- 1 large sweet potato, peeled and diced
- 1 tbsp olive oil
- 1/2 onion, diced
- 1 red bell pepper, diced
- 1 clove garlic, minced
- 2 cups of kale, stems removed and chopped
- Salt and pepper, to taste
- 1/2 tsp smoked paprika (optional)
- 2 large eggs (optional for serving)

Instructions

1. In a large skillet, heat the olive oil over medium heat.
2. Add the cubed sweet potato and simmer for 8-10 minutes, stirring periodically, until softened and browned.
3. Cook the onion, bell pepper, and garlic in the pan for another 5 minutes or until the onion is translucent and the veggies are cooked.
4. Add the chopped kale, season with salt, pepper, and smoked paprika (if using), and simmer for another 3-5 minutes, until the kale has wilted and everything is thoroughly mixed.
5. If using eggs, create two tiny wells in the hash, put an egg into each, cover the pan, and cook until the eggs are done to your preference.
6. Serve warm, with more seasoning as needed.

Nutrition Information (per serving, without eggs):

Calories: 200 Protein: 3 g Fat: 8 g Carbohydrates: 28 g Fiber: 6 g Sugar: 6 g

Ginger-Infused Greek Yogurt Parfait

Prep Time: 10 minutes

Servings: 2

Ingredients

- 1 cup of Greek yogurt
- 1/2 tsp fresh ginger, finely grated
- 1 tbsp honey or maple syrup (optional)
- 1/2 cup of granola
- 1/2 cup of mixed berries
- 1 tbsp chia seeds
- 1 tbsp chopped walnuts or almonds

Instructions

1. In a small bowl, blend the Greek yogurt, grated ginger, and honey or maple syrup, if using, until well combined.
2. In each serving glass or bowl, place 1/4 cup of ginger-infused yogurt, followed by granola, berries, and chia seeds.
3. Repeat layering with the remaining yogurt, granola, berries, and chia seeds.
4. To add crunch and texture, top each parfait with chopped nuts.
5. Serve immediately.

Nutrition Information (per serving):

Calories: 280 Protein: 12 g Fat: 10 g Carbohydrates: 36 g Fiber: 6 g Sugar: 14 g

Matcha Green Smoothie Bowl

Prep Time: 5 minutes

Servings: 2

Ingredients

- 1 cup of spinach leaves
- 1 banana, frozen and sliced
- 1/2 avocado
- 1/2 cup of unsweetened almond milk
- 1 tsp matcha green tea powder
- 1 tbsp chia seeds

Toppings:

- 1/4 cup of sliced strawberries
- 1/4 cup of granola
- 1 tbsp shredded coconut
- 1 tsp pumpkin seeds

Instructions

1. Add the spinach, frozen banana, avocado, almond milk, matcha powder, and chia seeds in a blender. Blend until smooth and creamy.
2. Pour the smoothie into two bowls.
3. Top each bowl with sliced strawberries, granola, shredded coconut, and pumpkin seeds for extra flavor and crunch.

Nutrition Information (per serving):

Calories: 300 Protein: 6 g Fat: 15 g Carbohydrates: 40 g Fiber: 9 g Sugar: 15 g

Almond Flour Protein Waffles

Prep Time: 10 minutes

Cook Time: 15 minutes

Servings: 4 waffles

Ingredients

- 1 cup of almond flour
- 1/4 cup of protein powder (vanilla or unflavored)
- 1 tsp baking powder
- 1/4 tsp salt
- 2 large eggs
- 1/4 cup of unsweetened almond milk
- 1 tbsp maple syrup or honey (optional)
- 1 tsp vanilla extract
- Coconut oil or cooking spray for greasing the waffle iron

Instructions

1. Preheat your waffle iron according to the manufacturer's directions, then gently coat it with coconut oil or cooking spray.
2. Combine almond flour, protein powder, baking powder, and salt in a large bowl.
3. Mix the eggs, almond milk, maple syrup, and vanilla extract in a second bowl until thoroughly combined.
4. Pour the wet ingredients into the dry ingredients and mix just until mixed. The batter will be thick.
5. Pour the batter onto the hot waffle iron (approximately 1/4 of the batter for each waffle) and fry for the recommended time, generally 3-5 minutes, until golden brown and cooked.
6. Serve warm.

Nutrition Information (per waffle):

Calories: 220 Protein: 12 g Fat: 16 g Carbohydrates: 8 g Fiber: 3 g Sugar: 2 g

Green Veggie Omelet

Prep Time: 5 minutes

Cook Time: 10 minutes

Servings: 1

Ingredients

- 2 large eggs
- 1 tbsp milk (any variety, optional)
- Salt and pepper, to taste
- 1 tsp olive oil or butter
- 1/4 cup of chopped spinach
- 1/4 cup of chopped zucchini
- 1/4 cup of chopped green bell pepper
- 1 tbsp chopped green onion
- 1 tbsp fresh parsley or cilantro, chopped (optional)

Instructions

1. Combine the eggs, milk, salt, and pepper in a mixing bowl and whisk thoroughly.
2. Heat the olive oil or butter in a nonstick pan over medium heat.
3. Add the spinach, zucchini, green bell pepper, and green onion to the skillet—Sauté for approximately 3 minutes or until the veggies are soft.
4. Pour the egg mixture over the vegetables in the skillet, turning it to ensure that the eggs are uniformly distributed.
5. Cook for 2-3 minutes, using a spatula to carefully raise the edges and allow any raw egg to seep beneath.
6. Once the eggs have nearly set, delicately fold the omelet in half. Cook for another minute until completely set.
7. Transfer the omelet to a plate and garnish with fresh parsley or cilantro.

Nutrition Information (per serving):

Calories: 180 Protein: 12 g Fat: 12 g Carbohydrates: 6 g Fiber: 2 g Sugar: 2 g

Raspberry Coconut Yogurt Bowl

Prep Time: 5 minutes

Servings: 1

Ingredients

- 1 cup of coconut yogurt
- 1/2 cup of fresh raspberries
- 1 tbsp unsweetened shredded coconut
- 1 tbsp chia seeds
- 1 tbsp sliced almonds or other nuts of choice
- 1 tsp honey or maple syrup (optional)

Instructions

1. In a serving bowl, place the coconut yogurt as the basis.
2. Garnish the yogurt with fresh raspberries, shredded coconut, chia seeds, and sliced almonds.
3. For a sweeter taste, drizzle with honey or maple syrup.
4. Serve immediately and enjoy!

Nutrition Information (per serving):

Calories: 250 Protein: 6 g Fat: 15 g Carbohydrates: 24 g Fiber: 8 g Sugar: 10 g

Cinnamon Apple Oatmeal Bake

Prep Time: 10 minutes

Cook Time: 35 minutes

Servings: 6

Ingredients

- 2 cups of rolled oats
- 1 1/2 tsp cinnamon
- 1/2 tsp nutmeg
- 1 tsp baking powder
- 1/4 tsp salt
- 1 1/2 cups of almond milk (or milk of choice)
- 1/4 cup of maple syrup or honey
- 2 large eggs
- 1 tsp vanilla extract
- 2 medium apples, peeled, cored, and diced
- 1/4 cup of chopped walnuts or pecans (optional)

Instructions

1. Preheat the oven to 350° Fahrenheit (175° Celsius). Grease or line an 8x8-inch baking dish with parchment paper.
2. Add rolled oats, cinnamon, nutmeg, baking powder, and salt in a large mixing bowl.
3. Mix the almond milk, maple syrup or honey, eggs, and vanilla extract in a separate bowl until smooth.
4. Pour the wet ingredients into the dry and stir until completely blended. Gently mix in the diced apples and nuts if using.
5. Pour the mixture into the prepared baking dish and distribute evenly.
6. Bake for 30–35 minutes until the top is brown and the oatmeal has set.
7. Allow it to cool for a few minutes before slicing and serving. Serve heated by itself or with a splash of milk.

Nutrition Information (per serving):

Calories: 220 Protein: 5 g Fat: 7 g Carbohydrates: 34 g Fiber: 5 g Sugar: 12 g

Spinach & Goat Cheese Breakfast Wrap

Prep Time: 5 minutes

Cook Time: 5 minutes

Servings: 1

Ingredients

- 1 whole-grain tortilla
- 2 large eggs
- Salt and pepper, to taste
- 1 tsp olive oil
- 1/2 cup of fresh spinach leaves
- 1/4 cup of crumbled goat cheese
- 1 tbsp chopped fresh herbs

Instructions

1. Mix the eggs, salt, and pepper in a small bowl.
2. Heat the olive oil in a nonstick skillet over medium heat. Add the spinach and simmer for about 1 minute or until wilted.
3. Pour the eggs over the spinach and heat, stirring gently, until scrambled and set (approximately 2-3 minutes).
4. Remove the pan from the heat and add the goat cheese, stirring until evenly distributed.
5. Place the tortilla on a flat surface, spoon the scrambled eggs and spinach mixture in the center, and top with fresh herbs if preferred.
6. Roll the tortilla firmly, tucking in the sides to make a wrap. Serve warm.

Nutrition Information (per serving):

Calories: 300 Protein: 15 g Fat: 18 g Carbohydrates: 20 g Fiber: 4 g Sugar: 2 g

Avocado & Berry Toast Duo

Prep Time: 5 minutes

Servings: 2 toasts

Ingredients

- 2 slices whole-grain or sourdough bread, toasted
- 1 ripe avocado
- 1/2 tsp lemon juice
- Salt and pepper, to taste
- 1/4 cup of mixed berries
- 1 tsp honey or maple syrup (optional)
- 1 tsp chia seeds

Instructions

1. Combine the avocado, lemon juice, salt, and pepper in a small mixing bowl until smooth.
2. Spread the mashed avocado equally on the two toasted bread pieces.
3. Top each slice with a handful of mixed berries, pushing them lightly into the avocado to hold them in place.
4. To add sweetness, drizzle a tiny quantity of honey or maple syrup over the berries.
5. If used, sprinkle with chia seeds to add more nutrients.
6. Serve immediately and enjoy.

Nutrition Information (per toast):

Calories: 200 Protein: 4 g Fat: 11 g Carbohydrates: 22 g Fiber: 6 g Sugar: 5 g

Spiced Sweet Potato Breakfast Muffins

Prep Time: 15 minutes Cook Time: 25 minutes Servings: 12 muffins

Ingredients

- 1 cup of mashed sweet potato
- 2 large eggs
- 1/4 cup of olive oil or melted coconut oil
- 1/4 cup of maple syrup or honey
- 1 tsp vanilla extract
- 1 cup of whole wheat flour
- 1/2 cup of almond flour
- 1 tsp baking powder
- 1/2 tsp baking soda
- 1 tsp cinnamon
- 1/2 tsp nutmeg
- 1/4 tsp ground ginger
- 1/4 tsp salt
- 1/4 cup of chopped walnuts or pecans (optional)

Instructions

1. Preheat the oven to 350°F (175° C). Line a muffin tray with paper liners or oil gently.
2. In a large mixing bowl, combine the mashed sweet potato, eggs, oil, maple syrup, and vanilla extract until smooth.
3. Mix the whole wheat flour, almond flour, baking powder, baking soda, cinnamon, nutmeg, crushed ginger, and salt in a separate bowl.
4. Gradually add the dry ingredients to the wet mixture, stirring only until mixed. Don't over-mix.
5. Fold in the chopped nuts, if desired. Divide the mixture evenly among the muffin cups, filling them approximately 3/4 full.
6. Bake for 20 to 25 minutes or until a toothpick inserted in the middle comes out clean.
7. Allow the muffins to cool in the tin for 5 minutes before transferring to a wire rack to finish cooling.

Nutrition Information (per muffin):

Calories: 150 Protein: 3 g Fat: 8 g Carbohydrates: 18 g Fiber: 3 g Sugar: 6 g

Quinoa Veggie Buddha Bowl

Prep Time: 15 minutes Cook Time: 25 minutes Serving: 2 servings

Ingredients

- 1 cup of quinoa, rinsed
- 2 cups of water
- 1 tbsp olive oil
- 1 small sweet potato, peeled and diced
- 1 cup of broccoli florets
- 1 red bell pepper, sliced
- 1/2 cup of shredded carrots
- 1/2 avocado, sliced
- 2 tbsp tahini
- 1 tbsp lemon juice
- 1 tsp maple syrup
- Salt and pepper to taste
- 1 tbsp sesame seeds (optional)
- Fresh parsley for garnish

Instructions

1. In a medium saucepan, bring 2 cups of water to a boil. Add the rinsed quinoa, turn the heat down low, and cover. Simmer for around 15 minutes or until the quinoa is fluffy and the water has been absorbed. Remove from the heat and fluff with a fork.
2. Preheat the oven to 400 °F (200 °C). Combine the diced sweet potatoes on a baking sheet with 1 tbsp olive oil, salt, and pepper. Spread them out in a single layer—roast for approximately 20 minutes, rotating halfway through, until soft and golden.
3. Steam the broccoli florets while the sweet potatoes bake for 5 minutes or until bright green and tender. Alternatively, sauté the broccoli in a pan with a little olive oil for a few minutes.
4. In a small mixing bowl, combine tahini, lemon juice, maple syrup, a sprinkle of salt, and water to thin it down. Adjust to your chosen consistency by adding additional water as needed.
5. Divide the cooked quinoa into two bowls. Place the roasted sweet potatoes, steamed broccoli, sliced bell pepper, shredded carrots, and avocado on top of the quinoa.

6. Pour the tahini dressing over the constructed bowl, then top with sesame seeds and fresh parsley for garnishes.
7. Serve immediately.

Nutrition (Per Serving):

Calories: 400 kcal Protein: 11g Carbohydrates: 50g Fat: 18g Fiber: 9g Sugars: 8g Sodium: 220mg

Turmeric-Cauliflower Rice Bowl

Prep Time: 10 minutes Cook Time: 15 minutes Serving: 2 servings

Ingredients

- 1 small head of cauliflower, grated or riced
- 1 tbsp olive oil
- 1/2 tsp turmeric powder
- 1/4 tsp cumin powder
- 1/4 tsp garlic powder
- Salt and pepper to taste
- 1 tbsp lemon juice
- 1/2 cup of chickpeas, cooked or canned, drained and rinsed
- 1/4 cup of chopped cucumber
- 1/4 cup of cherry tomatoes, halved
- 1/4 cup of red onion, thinly sliced
- 1 tbsp fresh cilantro, chopped
- 1/4 avocado, sliced
- 1 tbsp tahini (optional)

Instructions

1. Use a box grater or a food processor to shred the cauliflower into rice-sized pieces. In a large skillet, heat olive oil over medium heat. Add the cauliflower rice to the pan and cook for 5-7 minutes or until softened. Stir periodically to avoid scorching.
2. Once the cauliflower rice is soft, add the turmeric, cumin, garlic powder, salt, and pepper. Cook for 2-3 minutes, enabling the spices to permeate the cauliflower rice.
3. While the cauliflower rice cooks, prepare the toppings. In a small bowl, combine the chickpeas with a touch of salt and pepper. Set aside. Chop the cucumber, cherry tomatoes, and red onion. Slice the avocado for garnish.

4. When the cauliflower rice is cooked, transfer it to a bowl. Place the chickpeas, cucumber, tomatoes, red onion, and avocado on top of the cauliflower rice.
5. Drizzle the bowl with lemon juice and, if preferred, a spoonful of tahini to add smoothness. Garnish with fresh cilantro and more salt and pepper to taste.
6. Enjoy.

Nutrition (Per Serving):

Calories: 250 kcal Protein: 8g Carbohydrates: 22g Fat: 14g Fiber: 8g Sugars: 6g Sodium: 180mg

Grilled Salmon and Greens Salad

Prep Time: 15 minutes Cook Time: 10 minutes Serving: 2

Ingredients

- 2 salmon fillets (6 oz each)
- 1 tbsp olive oil
- 1 tsp lemon zest
- 1 tsp dried oregano
- Salt and pepper to taste
- 4 cups of mixed greens
- 1 cucumber, thinly sliced
- 1/2 red onion, thinly sliced
- 1 avocado, sliced
- 1 tbsp pumpkin seeds
- 1 tbsp olive oil (for dressing)
- 1 tbsp balsamic vinegar
- Juice of half a lemon
- 1 tsp Dijon mustard

Instructions

1. Preheat the grill to medium-high heat. Coat the salmon fillets with olive oil, lemon zest, oregano, salt, and pepper.
2. Place the salmon on the grill and cook for 3-4 minutes on each side until it readily flakes with the fork.
3. While the salmon is cooking, make the salad: In a large bowl, combine the mixed greens, cucumber, red onion, and avocado.

4. Mix olive oil, balsamic vinegar, lemon juice, and Dijon mustard in a small bowl to prepare the dressing.
5. After the salmon has been cooked, cut it into large slices and serve it over the salad. Drizzle the dressing over the salad, then top with pumpkin seeds for crunch.
6. Toss the salad lightly to mix, then serve immediately.

Nutrition (per serving):

Calories: 450 Protein: 30g Fat: 30g Carbohydrates: 10g Fiber: 6g Sugars: 3g Sodium: 350mg

Zucchini Noodle Bowl with Pesto

Prep Time: 15 minutes Cook Time: 5 minutes Serving: 2

Ingredients

- 2 medium zucchinis, spiralized into noodles
- 1 tbsp olive oil
- 1/2 cup of fresh basil leaves
- 2 tbsp pine nuts
- 1/4 cup of grated Parmesan cheese
- 1 garlic clove
- 1/4 cup of olive oil (for pesto)
- 1 tbsp lemon juice
- Salt and pepper to taste
- 1 tbsp cherry tomatoes, halved
- 1 tbsp pumpkin seeds

Instructions

1. In a large pan, heat 1 tbsp olive oil over medium heat.
2. Sauté the zucchini noodles for 2-3 minutes until soft yet al dente. Remove from the heat and put aside.
3. Make the pesto by combining basil, pine nuts, Parmesan (or nutritional yeast), garlic, olive oil, lemon juice, salt, and pepper in a food processor. Blend until smooth and creamy.
4. Toss the zucchini noodles in the prepared pesto until well-covered.
5. Divide the pesto zucchini noodles into two bowls. Garnish with halved cherry tomatoes and pumpkin seeds, if preferred.
6. Serve immediately and enjoy!

Nutrition (per serving):

Calories: 300 Protein: 7g Fat: 28g Carbohydrates: 12g Fiber: 4g Sugars: 6g Sodium: 180mg

Lentil & Beet Salad with Walnuts

Prep Time: 15 minutes Cook Time: 30 minutes Serving: 2

Ingredients

- 1 cup of dried green or brown lentils, rinsed
- 2 medium beets, roasted and peeled
- 1/2 red onion, thinly sliced
- 1/2 cup of walnuts, toasted and chopped
- 4 cups of mixed greens
- 1 tbsp olive oil (for dressing)
- 1 tbsp apple cider vinegar
- 1 tsp Dijon mustard
- 1 tbsp honey or maple syrup
- Salt and pepper to taste
- 1/4 tsp ground cumin (optional)
- 1/4 cup of crumbled feta cheese

Instructions

1. In a medium saucepan, bring 3 cups of water to a boil. Add the lentils, lower the heat to a simmer, and cook for 20-25 minutes or until cooked but firm. Drain and put aside.
2. While the lentils simmer, cover the beets in foil and bake in a preheated oven at 400°F (200°C) for 25-30 minutes or until soft. After roasting, peel the beets and chop them into tiny pieces.
3. In a small mixing bowl, combine the olive oil, apple cider vinegar, Dijon mustard, honey or maple syrup, cumin (if using), salt, and pepper to make the dressing.
4. Mix the cooked lentils, roasted beets, red onion, and greens in a large bowl.
5. Drizzle the dressing over the salad and gently toss to mix.
6. Sprinkle the toasted walnuts and crumbled feta (if using) over the top for extra crunch and flavor.
7. Serve immediately or chill in the fridge for 30 minutes to make a cooler salad.

Nutrition (per serving):

Calories: 380 Protein: 15g Fat: 20g Carbohydrates: 40g Fiber: 12g Sugars: 8g Sodium: 230mg

Spinach and Chickpea Curry Wrap

Prep Time: 10 minutes

Cook Time: 15 minutes

Serving: 2

Ingredients

- 1 tbsp olive oil
- 1 small onion, diced
- 2 garlic cloves, minced
- 1 tbsp grated fresh ginger
- 1 can (15 oz) chickpeas, drained and rinsed
- 2 cups of fresh spinach leaves, chopped
- 1/2 cup of canned diced tomatoes
- 1/4 cup of coconut milk
- 1 tbsp curry powder
- 1 tsp ground cumin
- 1/2 tsp ground turmeric
- Salt and pepper to taste
- 2 whole wheat or spinach wraps
- 1 tbsp cilantro, chopped (for garnish)
- 1 tbsp plain Greek yogurt (optional for topping)

Instructions

1. In a large pan, heat the olive oil over medium heat. Sauté the diced onion for 3-4 minutes, until softened.
2. Cook for another minute until the minced garlic and grated ginger are fragrant.
3. Combine the chickpeas, spinach, chopped tomatoes, coconut milk, curry powder, cumin, and turmeric. Cook for 5-7 minutes, stirring regularly, until the spinach wilts and the flavors combine.
4. Season with salt and pepper to taste.
5. Warm the wraps in a dry skillet for 1-2 minutes until soft and malleable. Spoon the chickpea curry into the middle of each wrap.
6. Garnish with chopped cilantro and a dollop of Greek yogurt if preferred. Fold the sides of the wrap and roll it tightly. Serve immediately.

Nutrition (per serving):

Calories: 350 Protein: 15g Fat: 18g Carbohydrates: 38g Fiber: 9g Sugars: 7g Sodium: 450mg

Miso-Glazed Tofu Bowl

Prep Time: 15 minutes Cook Time: 20 minutes Serving: 2

Ingredients

- 1 block (14 oz) firm tofu, pressed and cut into cubes
- 1 tbsp olive oil
- 2 tbsp miso paste
- 1 tbsp rice vinegar
- 1 tbsp maple syrup
- 1 tsp soy sauce
- 1 tsp sesame oil
- 1/2 tsp grated fresh ginger
- 1/2 cup of cooked quinoa (or brown rice)
- 1 cup of steamed broccoli florets
- 1/2 cup of shredded carrots
- 1/4 cup of sliced cucumber
- 1 tbsp sesame seeds
- 1 tbsp chopped green onions (optional)
- 1/2 avocado, sliced (optional)

Instructions

1. Preheat the oven to 400 °F (200 °C). Line a baking sheet with parchment paper.
2. Place the cubed tofu on a baking pan, spray with olive oil, and bake for 20 minutes, turning halfway, or until golden and crispy.
3. While the tofu is baking, combine the miso paste, rice vinegar, maple syrup, soy sauce, sesame oil, and grated ginger in a small mixing bowl.
4. Mix the cooked quinoa, steamed broccoli, shredded carrots, and sliced cucumber in a medium bowl.
5. When the tofu is done, take it from the oven and toss it in the miso glaze until well covered. Divide the quinoa and veggie mixture into two bowls and top with the glazed tofu.
6. Garnish with sesame seeds, chopped green onions, or sliced avocado if preferred.
7. Serve immediately and enjoy!

Nutrition (per serving):

Calories: 400 Protein: 18g Fat: 22g Carbohydrates: 35g Fiber: 8g Sugars: 12g Sodium: 750mg

Sweet Potato and Black Bean Tacos

Prep Time: 10 minutes Cook Time: 25 minutes Serving: 2

Ingredients

- 2 medium sweet potatoes, peeled and diced
- 1 tbsp olive oil
- 1 tsp ground cumin
- 1 tsp chili powder
- Salt and pepper to taste
- 1 can (15 oz) black beans, drained and rinsed
- 1/2 red onion, diced
- 1 avocado, sliced
- 4 small corn tortillas (or whole wheat)
- 1 tbsp fresh cilantro, chopped
- 1 tbsp lime juice
- 1/4 cup of crumbled feta cheese (optional)
- 1 tbsp salsa (optional for topping)

Instructions

1. Preheat the oven to 400 °F (200 °C). Line a baking sheet with parchment paper.
2. Mix the chopped sweet potatoes with olive oil, cumin, chili powder, salt, and pepper. Place them in a single layer on the baking sheet.
3. Roast for 20-25 minutes, rotating halfway through or until the sweet potatoes are soft and gently caramelized.
4. While the sweet potatoes are roasting, cook the black beans in a small skillet over medium heat, stirring occasionally until heated—season with salt and pepper to taste.
5. Warm the tortillas in a dry skillet for 1-2 minutes until they are soft and malleable.
6. When the sweet potatoes are finished, assemble the tacos: Spread a few spoonful of roasted sweet potatoes on each tortilla, then top with black beans, sliced red onion, and avocado slices.
7. Garnish with fresh cilantro, a squeeze of lime juice, and crumbled feta (optional). If you want more taste, add a tsp. of salsa.
8. Serve immediately and enjoy!

Nutrition (per serving):

Calories: 380 Protein: 12g Fat: 18g Carbohydrates: 48g Fiber: 12g Sugars: 12g Sodium: 450mg

Kale and Avocado Caesar Salad

Prep Time: 10 minutes

Cook Time: 5 minutes

Serving: 2

Ingredients

- 4 cups of kale, torn into bite-sized pieces
- One ripe avocado, peeled and sliced
- 1 tbsp olive oil (for sautéing)
- 1/4 cup of whole-grain croutons
- 1/4 cup of Parmesan cheese, shaved
- 1 tbsp lemon juice
- 2 tbsp tahini
- 1 tbsp apple cider vinegar
- 1 tbsp Dijon mustard
- 1 tsp garlic powder
- 1/2 tsp ground black pepper
- Salt to taste
- 1 tbsp water (to thin dressing, as needed)

Instructions

1. Massage the kale leaves in a large bowl with olive oil for 1-2 minutes to soften. This reduces the bitterness and makes the kale softer.
2. While massaging the greens, make the dressing. Combine tahini, lemon juice, apple cider vinegar, Dijon mustard, garlic powder, black pepper, and a sprinkle of salt in a small mixing bowl. Add water gradually until the dressing has a creamy, pourable consistency.
3. Toss the avocado pieces into the greens until evenly distributed.
4. Drizzle the dressing over the kale and avocado, swirling until evenly covered.
5. Sprinkle shaved Parmesan cheese on top, followed by croutons for crunch.
6. Serve immediately as a light, refreshing main course or side salad.

Nutrition (per serving):

Calories: 350 Protein: 8g Fat: 27g Carbohydrates: 22g Fiber: 9g Sugars: 4g Sodium: 450mg

Broccoli and Almond Salad

Prep Time: 10 minutes

Cook Time: 5 minutes

Serving: 2

Ingredients

- 2 cups of broccoli florets, steamed or blanched
- 1/4 cup of almonds, sliced or slivered
- 1/4 cup of red bell pepper, diced
- 1 tbsp olive oil
- 1 tbsp apple cider vinegar
- 1 tsp Dijon mustard
- 1 tsp honey or maple syrup
- 1/4 tsp garlic powder
- Salt and pepper to taste
- 1 tbsp fresh parsley, chopped (for garnish)
- 1 tbsp sunflower seeds

Instructions

1. Steam or blanch the broccoli florets for 3-4 minutes until soft but still brilliant green. Drain, then put aside to cool somewhat.
2. While the broccoli cools, toast the almonds in a dry pan over medium heat for 2-3 minutes, tossing often until golden brown and aromatic. Remove from the heat and put aside.
3. In a small mixing bowl, combine olive oil, apple cider vinegar, Dijon mustard, honey or maple syrup, garlic powder, salt, and pepper to make the dressing.
4. Add steamed broccoli, roasted almonds, and chopped red bell pepper in a large mixing bowl.
5. Drizzle the dressing over the salad, tossing carefully to cover all ingredients.
6. For extra crunch and taste, garnish with fresh parsley and, if desired, sunflower seeds.
7. Serve immediately.

Nutrition (per serving):

Calories: 250 Protein: 8g Fat: 20g Carbohydrates: 18g Fiber: 8g Sugars: 6g Sodium: 220mg

Curried Cauliflower & Quinoa Bowl

Prep Time: 15 minutes

Cook Time: 25 minutes

Servings: 2

Ingredients

- 1/2 cup of quinoa, rinsed
- 1 cup of water
- 1/2 head cauliflower, cut into florets
- 1 tbsp olive oil
- 1/2 tsp ground turmeric
- 1/2 tsp ground cumin
- 1/2 tsp ground coriander
- 1/4 tsp ground cinnamon
- 1/2 tsp sea salt, divided
- 1 cup of baby spinach
- 1/4 cup of chopped cilantro for garnish
- 1/4 cup of pumpkin seeds, toasted
- 1/2 avocado, sliced
- 1 tbsp lemon juice (for drizzling)

Instructions

1. In a medium saucepan, heat the quinoa and water until boiling. Reduce the heat, cover, and let it simmer for approximately 15 minutes, or until the quinoa has absorbed the water and become fluffy. Set aside.
2. Preheat the oven to 400 °F (200 °C). Place the cauliflower florets on a baking sheet, drizzle with olive oil, and season with turmeric, cumin, coriander, cinnamon, and 1/4 tsp salt. Toss to coat—Roast for 20 to 25 minutes or until the cauliflower is soft and gently browned.
3. Divide the cooked quinoa into two bowls. Top each bowl with roasted cauliflower, spinach, chopped cilantro, toasted pumpkin seeds, and avocado slices.
4. Drizzle lemon juice into each bowl and add the remaining salt. Serve warm and enjoy!

Nutrition (per serving)

Calories: 320 Protein: 10g Carbohydrates: 36g Fiber: 11g Fat: 17g

Detox Veggie Stir-Fry

Prep Time: 10 minutes

Cook Time: 15 minutes

Servings: 2

Ingredients

- 1 tbsp coconut oil
- 1/2 red onion, thinly sliced
- 1 red bell pepper, thinly sliced
- 1 cup of broccoli florets
- 1 cup of carrots, julienned or thinly sliced
- 1/2 cup of snow peas, trimmed
- 1/2 tsp grated ginger
- 2 cloves garlic, minced
- 1 tbsp coconut aminos (or low-sodium soy sauce)
- 1 tbsp fresh lemon juice
- 1/2 tsp turmeric powder
- 1/4 tsp ground black pepper
- 1/4 cup of fresh cilantro, chopped (for garnish)
- 1 tbsp sesame seeds (optional, for garnish)

Instructions

1. Heat the coconut oil in a large pan or wok over medium heat. Stir in the sliced onion and simmer for 2 minutes or until softened.
2. Increase the heat to medium-high, then add the red bell pepper, broccoli, carrots, and snow peas. Stir-fry for 5-7 minutes until the veggies are soft and crisp.
3. Add the grated ginger, minced garlic, coconut aminos, lemon juice, turmeric, and black pepper to the skillet. Stir well to mix, then heat for 2-3 minutes until everything is coated and aromatic.
4. Remove from heat. Sprinkle with fresh cilantro and sesame seeds if preferred. Serve warm.

Nutrition (per serving)

Calories: 180 Protein: 4g Carbohydrates: 22g Fiber: 7g Fat: 9g

Mediterranean Hummus Bowl

Prep Time: 10 minutes

Cook Time: 0 minutes

Servings: 2

Ingredients

- 1 cup of hummus (store-bought or homemade)
- 1/2 cup of cherry tomatoes, halved
- 1/2 cucumber, sliced
- 1/4 cup of red onion, thinly sliced
- 1/4 cup of Kalamata olives, pitted and halved
- 1/4 cup of roasted red peppers, sliced
- 1 tbsp extra virgin olive oil
- 1 tbsp lemon juice
- 1/2 tsp dried oregano
- 1/4 tsp sea salt
- 1/4 tsp black pepper
- 1 tbsp fresh parsley, chopped (for garnish)
- 1 tbsp pine nuts, toasted (optional, for garnish)

Instructions

1. Divide the hummus equally between two bowls, making an even layer at each bottom.
2. Place cherry tomatoes, cucumber slices, red onion, olives, and roasted red peppers in each bowl on top of the hummus.
3. Drizzle olive oil and lemon juice over the vegetables. Season with oregano, salt, and black pepper.
4. Garnish with fresh parsley and toasted pine nuts for added crunch. Serve immediately with whole grain pita or as a light meal.

Nutrition (per serving)

Calories: 280 Protein: 8g Carbohydrates: 28g Fiber: 7g Fat: 18g Vitamin C: 25mg Magnesium: 60mg

Grilled Lemon Chicken Salad

Prep Time: 15 minutes

Cook Time: 10 minutes

Servings: 2

Ingredients

- 2 boneless, skinless chicken breasts
- 1 tbsp olive oil
- Juice of 1 lemon
- 1 clove garlic, minced
- 1 tsp dried oregano
- 1/2 tsp sea salt
- 1/4 tsp black pepper
- 4 cups of mixed salad greens
- 1/2 cucumber, sliced
- 1/2 cup of cherry tomatoes, halved
- 1/4 red onion, thinly sliced
- 1/4 cup of feta cheese, crumbled (optional)
- 1 tbsp fresh parsley, chopped (for garnish)

Instructions

1. Add olive oil, lemon juice, minced garlic, oregano, salt, and pepper in a small mixing bowl. Place the chicken breasts in a resealable bag or shallow bowl, pour the marinade over them, and refrigerate for at least 15 minutes (or up to an hour) to enable the flavors to combine.
2. Preheat the grill or grill pan to medium-high heat. Grill the chicken for 4-5 minutes on each side or until fully cooked, reaching an internal temperature of 165°F (75°C). Remove off the grill and let cool for a few minutes before slicing thinly.
3. While the chicken rests, combine the salad greens, cucumber, cherry tomatoes, and red onion in a large bowl or individual plates.
4. Top the salad with the grilled chicken slices. Add crumbled feta cheese and sprinkle with fresh parsley.
5. Drizzle with more olive oil and lemon juice if preferred, and serve immediately.

Nutrition (per serving)

Calories: 350 Protein: 35g Carbohydrates: 12g Fiber: 4g Fat: 18g

Herb-Roasted Root Vegetable Bowl

Prep Time: 10 minutes

Cook Time: 30 minutes

Servings: 2

Ingredients

- 1 medium sweet potato, peeled and cubed
- 2 carrots, peeled and sliced
- 1 parsnip, peeled and sliced
- 1 small red onion, cut into wedges
- 1 tbsp olive oil
- 1 tsp dried thyme
- 1 tsp dried rosemary
- 1/2 tsp garlic powder
- 1/2 tsp sea salt
- 1/4 tsp black pepper
- 2 cups of mixed greens
- 1 tbsp balsamic vinegar
- 1 tbsp pumpkin seeds (optional for topping)

Instructions

1. Preheat the oven to 400 °F (200 °C). Line a baking sheet with parchment paper.
2. Place the sweet potatoes, carrots, parsnips, and red onion on a baking sheet. Drizzle olive oil and season with thyme, rosemary, garlic powder, salt, and pepper. Toss everything until uniformly coated.
3. Roast the veggies for 25-30 minutes or until soft and lightly browned, tossing halfway through to ensure equal cooking.
4. Once the veggies have been roasted, take them from the oven and allow them to cool somewhat. Divide the mixed greens into two bowls. Top with the roasted veggies.
5. Drizzle with balsamic vinegar and top with pumpkin seeds, if desired. Serve warm.

Nutrition (per serving)

Calories: 280 Protein: 5g Carbohydrates: 40g Fiber: 9g Fat: 12g

Asian Ginger Salad Wraps

Prep Time: 15 minutes Cook Time: 0 minutes Servings: 2

Ingredients

- 4 large lettuce leaves
- 1/2 cup of shredded cabbage (green or purple)
- 1/2 cup of shredded carrots
- 1/2 cucumber, julienned
- 1/4 cup of red bell pepper, thinly sliced
- 1/4 cup of fresh cilantro, chopped
- 1/4 cup of green onions, thinly sliced
- 1 tbsp sesame seeds (optional)
- 1/2 cup of cooked chicken breast, shredded or sliced

For the Dressing:

- 2 tbsp tamari or coconut aminos
- 1 tbsp rice vinegar
- 1 tbsp fresh ginger, grated
- 1 tsp sesame oil
- 1 tsp honey or maple syrup (optional)
- 1/4 tsp garlic powder
- 1/4 tsp ground black pepper

Instructions

Add the shredded cabbage, carrots, julienned cucumber, red bell pepper, cilantro, and green onions in a medium mixing bowl. Toss lightly to combine.

In a small bowl, mix the tamari (or coconut aminos), rice vinegar, grated ginger, sesame oil, honey or maple syrup (if using), garlic powder, and black pepper until thoroughly blended.

Arrange the lettuce leaves flat on a clean surface. Place a large quantity of salad mixture in the middle of each leaf.

Drizzle some ginger dressing over the salad mixture in each lettuce leaf. If you're adding chicken or another protein, put it on top.

Carefully fold the lettuce leaves' edges over the filling and roll them up to form a wrap. Sprinkle with sesame seeds, if preferred. Serve immediately.

Nutrition (per serving)

Calories: 180 Protein: 6g (with chicken) Carbohydrates: 15g Fiber: 4g Fat: 12g

Zesty Shrimp and Avocado Salad

Prep Time: 15 minutes Cook Time: 5 minutes Servings: 2

Ingredients

- 8 oz cooked shrimp, peeled and deveined
- 1 large avocado, diced
- 2 cups of mixed greens
- 1/2 cup of cherry tomatoes, halved
- 1/4 cup of cucumber, sliced
- 1/4 cup of red onion, thinly sliced
- 1 tbsp fresh cilantro, chopped (for garnish)
- For the Dressing:
- 2 tbsp olive oil
- 1 tbsp fresh lime juice
- 1 tsp Dijon mustard
- 1/2 tsp chili powder
- 1/4 tsp sea salt
- 1/4 tsp black pepper
- 1/2 tsp honey (optional)

Instructions

1. Add the mixed greens, cherry tomatoes, cucumber, red onion, and cubed avocado in a large bowl. Toss lightly to combine.
2. In a small mixing bowl, combine the olive oil, lime juice, Dijon mustard, chili powder, salt, pepper, and honey (if using) until smooth and thoroughly blended.
3. Add the cooked shrimp to the salad and cover with the dressing. Gently toss everything together until coated.
4. Garnish with fresh cilantro and serve immediately.

Nutrition (per serving)

Calories: 280 Protein: 22g Carbohydrates: 12g Fiber: 6g Fat: 18g

Spicy Chickpea and Spinach Stew

Prep Time: 10 minutes Cook Time: 25 minutes Servings: 2

Ingredients

- 1 tbsp olive oil
- 1 small onion, chopped
- 2 cloves garlic, minced
- 1 tsp ground cumin
- 1/2 tsp ground turmeric
- 1/2 tsp ground paprika
- 1/4 tsp cayenne pepper
- 1 can (15 oz) chickpeas, drained and rinsed
- 1 can (14 oz) diced tomatoes with juice
- 2 cups of fresh spinach, packed
- 1/2 cup of vegetable broth (or water)
- 1 tbsp lemon juice
- Salt and pepper, to taste
- Fresh cilantro for garnish (optional)

Instructions

1. In a large saucepan, warm the olive oil over medium heat. Cook the chopped onion for 3-4 minutes, until tender and transparent. Add the minced garlic and simmer for another minute until fragrant.
2. Combine the cumin, turmeric, paprika, and cayenne pepper (if using). Cook for 1-2 minutes, stirring often, until the spices become fragrant.
3. Stir in the chickpeas and chopped tomatoes (with juice). Bring the mixture to a boil, then cook for 10-15 minutes, stirring regularly.
4. Add the fresh spinach once the chickpeas are soft and the flavors have combined. Stir until the spinach has wilted down.
5. Pour vegetable broth (or water) to get the desired stew consistency. Add the lemon juice and season with salt and pepper to taste.
6. Remove from heat. Ladle the stew into bowls and top with fresh cilantro, if preferred. Serve hot.

Nutrition (per serving)

Calories: 250 Protein: 12g Carbohydrates: 38g Fiber: 10g Fat: 8g

Ginger Sesame Salmon

Prep Time: 10 minutes

Cook Time: 15 minutes

Servings: 2

Ingredients

- 2 salmon fillets (6 oz each)
- 1 tbsp sesame oil
- 1 tbsp fresh ginger, grated
- 2 tbsp tamari or coconut aminos
- 1 tbsp honey or maple syrup (optional)
- 1 tbsp rice vinegar
- 1 clove garlic, minced
- 1/2 tsp sesame seeds, toasted
- 1/2 tsp chili flakes (optional, for spice)
- 1 green onion, sliced (for garnish)
- Lime wedges for serving

Instructions

1. Combine sesame oil, grated ginger, tamari (or coconut aminos), honey, rice vinegar, and chopped garlic in a small mixing bowl.
2. Place the salmon fillets in a shallow bowl and pour the marinade. Allow at least 10 minutes for the flavors to seep in.
3. Preheat a nonstick skillet or grill pan to medium-high heat. Once heated, add the salmon fillets, skin side down, and cook for 4-5 minutes on each side until the salmon is cooked through and easily flaked with a fork.
4. When the salmon has been cooked, sprinkle any leftover marinade over the fillets. Garnish with toasted sesame seeds and chili flakes (if desired). Garnish with sliced green onions.
5. Serve immediately.

Nutrition (per serving)

Calories: 320 Protein: 25g Carbohydrates: 8g Fiber: 2g Fat: 22g

Stuffed Bell Peppers with Quinoa and Veggies

Prep Time: 15 minutes

Cook Time: 30 minutes

Servings: 2

Ingredients

- 2 large bell peppers, any color
- 1/2 cup of quinoa, rinsed
- 1 cup of water or vegetable broth
- 1 tbsp olive oil
- 1 small onion, chopped
- 1/2 cup of zucchini, diced
- 1/2 cup of cherry tomatoes, chopped
- 1/4 cup of corn kernels (fresh or frozen)
- 1/4 cup of black beans, drained and rinsed (optional)
- 1 tsp ground cumin
- 1/2 tsp paprika
- 1/4 tsp ground black pepper
- 1/2 tsp sea salt
- 1/4 cup of fresh cilantro, chopped
- 1 tbsp lime juice
- 1/4 cup of crumbled feta or goat cheese (optional for topping)

Instructions

1. Heat the quinoa and water (or vegetable broth) in a small saucepan until boiling. Reduce the heat, cover, and let it simmer for approximately 15 minutes or until the quinoa is cooked and fluffy. Set aside.
2. While the quinoa is cooking, prepare the oven to 375°F (190°C). Cut off the tops of the bell peppers and remove the seeds. Place the peppers in a baking dish upright.
3. In a medium-sized pan, heat the olive oil over medium heat. Sauté the chopped onion for 3-4 minutes, until tender. Combine the zucchini, cherry tomatoes, corn, and black beans (if using). Cook for 5-7 minutes until the veggies are soft. Season with cumin, paprika, black pepper, and salt.
4. Add the cooked quinoa, sautéed veggies, chopped cilantro, and lime juice in a large mixing bowl. Stir until well blended.
5. Spoon the quinoa mixture into each bell pepper, packing it carefully. To add flavor, sprinkle the tops with crumbled feta or goat cheese.

6. Cover the baking dish with foil and bake for 20-25 minutes or until the peppers are soft. Remove the foil during the last 5 minutes of baking to let the cheese melt and color.

7. Remove the peppers from the oven and serve immediately, with more cilantro as desired.

Nutrition (per serving)

Calories: 280 Protein: 10g Carbohydrates: 45g Fiber: 8g Fat: 9g

Lentil & Vegetable Shepherd's Pie

Prep Time: 15 minutes Cook Time: 40 minutes Servings: 4

Ingredients

- For the filling:
- 1 tbsp olive oil
- 1 small onion, chopped
- 2 cloves garlic, minced
- 1 cup of carrots, diced
- 1 cup of celery, diced
- 1 cup of mushrooms, sliced
- 1 cup of green or brown lentils, cooked
- 1 can (14 oz) diced tomatoes with juice
- 1/2 cup of vegetable broth
- 1 tbsp tomato paste
- 1 tsp dried thyme
- 1/2 tsp ground cumin
- 1/2 tsp paprika
- Salt and pepper, to taste
- For the mashed potatoes:
- 3 medium potatoes, peeled and chopped
- 1 tbsp olive oil (or vegan butter)
- 1/4 cup of unsweetened almond milk (or any plant-based milk)
- 1/2 tsp sea salt
- 1/4 tsp black pepper

Instructions

1. Put the chopped potatoes in a saucepan and cover with water. Bring to a boil, then simmer for 10-15 minutes or until tender. Drain the potatoes and return them to the saucepan. Combine olive oil (or vegan butter), almond milk, salt, and pepper. Mash until smooth and creamy. Set aside.
2. While the potatoes simmer, warm the olive oil in a large pan over medium heat. Cook the onion and garlic for 3-4 minutes or until softened.
3. Add the chopped carrots, celery, and mushrooms to the skillet. Cook for a further 5-7 minutes until the veggies soften.
4. Combine the cooked lentils, diced tomatoes, vegetable broth, tomato paste, thyme, cumin, and paprika. Bring the mixture to a simmer and cook for 10 minutes, stirring regularly, until the flavors have blended and the sauce thickens. Season with salt and pepper to taste.
5. Preheat the oven to 375°F (190° C). Transfer the lentil and veggie mixture to a baking dish. Spread the mashed potatoes evenly over the filling, smoothing the surface with a spoon.
6. Place the baking dish in the oven for 15-20 minutes or until the top is brown and crispy.
7. Remove from the oven and let it cool for a few minutes before serving.

Nutrition (per serving)

Calories: 320 Protein: 14g Carbohydrates: 50g Fiber: 10g Fat: 8g

Garlic-Roasted Sweet Potato & Broccoli

Prep Time: 10 minutes

Cook Time: 30 minutes

Servings: 2

Ingredients

- 2 medium sweet potatoes, peeled and cubed
- 2 cups of broccoli florets
- 2 tbsp olive oil
- 4 cloves garlic, minced
- 1/2 tsp ground cumin
- 1/2 tsp paprika
- 1/4 tsp ground black pepper
- 1/2 tsp sea salt
- 1 tbsp fresh parsley, chopped (for garnish)
- 1 tbsp lemon juice (optional)

Instructions

1. Preheat the oven to 400 °F (200 °C). Line a baking sheet with parchment paper for easy cleaning.
2. Put the cubed sweet potatoes and broccoli florets on a baking sheet. Drizzle with olive oil and season with minced garlic, cumin, paprika, black pepper, and salt. Toss everything together until evenly coated.
3. Roast in a preheated oven for 25-30 minutes, stirring halfway through, until the sweet potatoes are soft and slightly caramelized and the broccoli is crisp.
4. After roasting, remove the veggies from the oven and sprinkle with fresh lemon juice. Garnish with chopped parsley before serving.

Nutrition (per serving)

Calories: 230 Protein: 5g Carbohydrates: 45g Fiber: 9g Fat: 8g

Lemon & Herb Baked Chicken

Prep Time: 10 minutes

Cook Time: 30 minutes

Servings: 2

Ingredients

- 2 boneless, skinless chicken breasts (about 6 oz each)
- 2 tbsp olive oil
- Juice of 1 lemon
- Zest of 1 lemon
- 2 cloves garlic, minced
- 1 tsp dried thyme
- 1 tsp dried rosemary
- 1/2 tsp sea salt
- 1/4 tsp black pepper
- 1 tbsp fresh parsley, chopped (for garnish)

Instructions

1. Mix olive oil, lemon juice, lemon zest, minced garlic, dried thyme, rosemary, salt, and black pepper in a small bowl. Whisk until well blended.
2. Place the chicken breasts in a shallow bowl or sealable bag. Pour the marinade over the chicken, ensuring it's well covered. Refrigerate for at least 10 minutes (or up to 2 hours) to let the flavors combine.
3. Preheat the oven to 375°F (190° C). Place the marinated chicken breasts on a baking sheet covered with parchment paper or in a baking dish. Bake for 25-30 minutes, or until the chicken is well cooked and has reached an internal temperature of 165°F (75°C).
4. Remove from the oven and let the chicken rest for a few minutes before slicing. Garnish with fresh parsley and serve.

Nutrition (per serving)

Calories: 270 Protein: 30g Carbohydrates: 2g Fiber: 1g Fat: 17g

Zucchini and Eggplant Lasagna

Prep Time: 15 minutes Cook Time: 40 minutes Servings: 4

Ingredients

- 2 medium zucchini, sliced lengthwise into thin strips
- 2 medium eggplants, sliced lengthwise into thin strips
- 1 tbsp olive oil
- 2 cups of ricotta cheese
- 1 1/2 cups of marinara sauce
- 1 cup of fresh spinach, chopped
- 1/2 cup of fresh basil, chopped
- 1/4 cup of nutritional yeast
- 1 tbsp dried oregano
- 1/2 tsp sea salt
- 1/4 tsp black pepper
- 1 cup of shredded mozzarella (or dairy-free cheese)

Instructions

1. Preheat the oven to 375° Fahrenheit (190° Celsius). Place the zucchini and eggplant slices on a baking sheet lined with parchment paper. Drizzle with olive oil and a bit of salt. Roast the veggies in the oven for 20-25 minutes, turning halfway through, until soft and lightly browned. Set aside.
2. In a medium mixing bowl, combine the ricotta, chopped spinach, basil, nutritional yeast (if using), oregano, salt, and pepper. Stir until well combined.
3. Cover the bottom of a 9x9-inch baking dish with a thin coating of marinara sauce. Layer with roasted zucchini slices, eggplant slices, ricotta mixture, and more marinara sauce. Repeat the layers until all ingredients have been utilized, ending with a layer of sauce on top.
4. Sprinkle the shredded mozzarella on top of the sauce.
5. Cover the baking dish with foil and bake for 25 to 30 minutes. Remove the foil and bake for 10 minutes or until the top is golden and bubbling.
6. Allow lasagna to cool for a few minutes before slicing. Garnish with fresh basil if preferred, and serve warm.

Nutrition (per serving)

Calories: 250 Protein: 14g Carbohydrates: 18g Fiber: 6g Fat: 16g

Roasted Cauliflower Steaks with Tahini Sauce

Prep Time: 10 minutes Cook Time: 30 minutes Servings: 2

Ingredients

- 1 large head of cauliflower, sliced into 1-inch thick steaks
- 2 tbsp olive oil
- 1/2 tsp ground cumin
- 1/2 tsp paprika
- 1/4 tsp sea salt
- 1/4 tsp black pepper
- 1 tbsp fresh parsley, chopped (for garnish)
- For the Tahini Sauce:
- 3 tbsp tahini
- 1 tbsp lemon juice
- 1 tbsp olive oil
- 1 clove garlic, minced
- 2 tbsp water (or more to thin)
- 1/4 tsp sea salt
- 1/4 tsp black pepper

Instructions

1. Preheat the oven to 400 °F (200 °C). Line a baking sheet with parchment paper.
2. Remove the cauliflower's outer leaves and cut the stem to stand flat. Cut the cauliflower into 1-inch thick steaks. Drizzle olive oil over both sides of the steaks and season with cumin, paprika, salt, and black pepper.
3. Place the cauliflower steaks on the prepared baking sheet. Roast in a preheated oven for 25-30 minutes, turning halfway through, or until golden brown and tender.
4. While the cauliflower roasts, add the tahini, lemon juice, olive oil, chopped garlic, water, salt, and pepper in a small bowl. Whisk until smooth, then add water for a creamy yet pourable consistency.
5. When the cauliflower steaks are done, remove them from the oven. Drizzle with tahini sauce and serve with chopped parsley.
6. Serve warm.

Nutrition (per serving)

Calories: 250 Protein: 7g Carbohydrates: 18g Fiber: 7g Fat: 18g

Herb-crusted tofu with Roasted Veggies

Prep Time: 15 minutes Cook Time: 30 minutes Servings: 2

Ingredients

- 1 block (14 oz) firm tofu, drained and pressed
- 2 tbsp olive oil
- 1 tsp dried oregano
- 1 tsp dried thyme
- 1/2 tsp garlic powder
- 1/2 tsp onion powder
- 1/4 tsp sea salt
- 1/4 tsp black pepper
- 1 tbsp nutritional yeast (optional for extra flavor)
- 1 small zucchini, sliced
- 1 bell pepper, chopped
- 1/2 cup of cherry tomatoes, halved
- 1 small red onion, sliced
- 1 tbsp olive oil
- 1/2 tsp ground cumin
- 1/2 tsp smoked paprika
- 1/4 tsp sea salt
- 1/4 tsp black pepper

Instructions

1. Preheat the oven to 400 °F (200 °C). Line two baking pans with parchment paper.
2. Cut the tofu into 1/2-inch pieces. To remove any extra moisture, dry each slice with a paper towel. Mix olive oil, oregano, thyme, garlic powder, onion powder, salt, pepper, and nutritional yeast (if using). Brush the herb mixture on both sides of the tofu pieces.
3. Place the zucchini, bell pepper, cherry tomatoes, and red onion on a baking sheet. Drizzle with olive oil, then season with cumin, smoked paprika, salt, and pepper. Toss the vegetables until uniformly coated.
4. Arrange the tofu pieces on the second baking sheet. Roast the tofu and vegetables in a warm oven for 25-30 minutes, turning midway through, until the tofu is golden and crispy and the vegetables are soft and slightly caramelized.
5. Once everything has been roasted, take it from the oven and place it on a platter. Serve the herb-crusted tofu with the roasted vegetables for a tasty meal.

Nutrition (per serving)

Calories: 350 Protein: 22g Carbohydrates: 30g Fiber: 10g Fat: 20g

Sweet Potato and Black Bean Enchiladas

Prep Time: 20 minutes Cook Time: 30 minutes Servings: 4

Ingredients

- 2 large sweet potatoes, peeled and diced
- 1 tbsp olive oil
- Salt and pepper, to taste
- 1 can (15 ounces) black beans, drained and rinsed
- 1 tsp ground cumin
- 1/2 tsp chili powder
- 1/4 tsp garlic powder
- 2 cups of enchilada sauce
- 8 whole wheat tortillas
- 1 cup of shredded cheese (optional for topping)
- Fresh cilantro, chopped (for garnish)
- Avocado slices (for serving)

Instructions

1. Preheat the oven to 400 °F (200 °C). Toss the diced sweet potatoes with olive oil, salt, and pepper on a baking sheet. Roast in the oven for about 20 minutes or until tender.
2. Combine the roasted sweet potatoes, black beans, cumin, chili powder, and garlic powder in a bowl. Stir until well blended.
3. Pour approximately 1/2 cup of enchilada sauce into the bottom of a baking dish.
4. Warm the tortillas slightly to make them pliable. Spread the sweet potato and bean mixture equally on each tortilla. Roll the tortillas and set the seam side down in the baking dish.
5. Pour the leftover enchilada sauce over the rolled tortillas, covering them thoroughly.
6. If using, sprinkle the top with shredded cheese. Bake for about 10 minutes or until the cheese is melted and bubbling.
7. Serve hot.

Nutrition Details (per serving):

Calories: 350 Protein: 10g Fat: 10g Carbohydrates: 55g Fiber: 10g

Sweet Potato and Black Bean Enchiladas

Prep Time: 15 minutes Cook Time: 40 minutes Servings: 4

Ingredients

- 2 medium sweet potatoes, peeled and diced
- 1 can (15 oz) black beans, drained and rinsed
- 1 small red onion, diced
- 1 red bell pepper, diced
- 1 tsp olive oil
- 1 tsp cumin powder
- 1 tsp smoked paprika
- Salt and pepper, to taste
- 1/4 cup of fresh cilantro, chopped
- 1 can (15 oz) tomato sauce
- 1 tsp chili powder
- 1/2 tsp garlic powder
- 1/2 tsp onion powder
- 1/2 tsp dried oregano
- Salt and pepper, to taste
- 8 small whole-wheat or corn tortillas
- 1/2 cup of shredded dairy-free or regular cheese (optional)
- Fresh cilantro and sliced avocado for garnish

Instructions

1. Preheat the oven to 375° Fahrenheit (190° Celsius). In a large skillet, heat the olive oil over medium heat. Add the sweet potatoes and simmer for approximately 10 minutes, stirring periodically, until softened.
2. Cook for 5 minutes or until the red onion and bell pepper are soft. Add the black beans, cumin, smoked paprika, salt, and pepper, and mix thoroughly. Allow the filling to simmer for 2 minutes before removing it from the heat and stirring it in the fresh cilantro.
3. Mix the tomato sauce, chili powder, garlic powder, onion powder, and oregano in a small saucepan season with salt and pepper. Simmer on low heat for 5 minutes, then remove from heat.
4. Spread a tiny sauce on the bottom of a 9x13-inch baking dish. Lay approximately 1/4 cup of filling in each tortilla, fold it, and lay it seam-side down in the baking dish. Repeat for the remaining tortillas.

5. Pour the enchilada sauce over the rolled tortillas and distribute it evenly. If using, sprinkle with cheese.
6. Cover the dish with foil and bake for 20 minutes. Remove the cover and bake for 5 minutes or until the cheese melts and the sauce bubbles.
7. Before serving, garnish with chopped fresh cilantro and sliced avocado.

Nutrition (per serving)

Calories: 350 Protein: 10g Carbohydrates: 55g Fat: 10g Fiber: 12g

Moroccan Chickpea and Spinach Stew

Prep Time: 10 minutes Cook Time: 30 minutes Servings: 4

Ingredients

- 1 tbsp olive oil
- 1 medium onion, chopped
- 3 garlic cloves, minced
- 1 tsp ground cumin
- 1 tsp ground coriander
- 1/2 tsp ground cinnamon
- 1/4 tsp ground turmeric
- 1/4 tsp cayenne pepper (optional, for heat)
- 1 can (15 oz) diced tomatoes with juices
- 1 can (15 oz) chickpeas, drained and rinsed
- 4 cups of fresh spinach
- 2 cups of vegetable broth
- Salt and pepper, to taste
- 1/4 cup of fresh cilantro or parsley, chopped, for garnish
- Lemon wedges for serving

Instructions

1. In a large saucepan, heat the olive oil over medium heat. Add the onion and simmer for 5 minutes or until tender. Stir in the garlic and simmer for another minute.
2. Combine the cumin, coriander, cinnamon, turmeric, and cayenne pepper (if using). Stir the spices for one minute to unleash their scent.
3. Pour in the chopped tomatoes, their juices, and the vegetable broth. Bring the mixture to a boil, then cook for 5 minutes, stirring regularly.

4. Add the chickpeas and spinach to the saucepan, stirring until the spinach wilts and incorporates into the stew. If using frozen spinach, cook for an extra 5 minutes.
5. Reduce the heat and simmer the stew for 15 minutes. Season with salt and pepper to taste.
6. Ladle the stew into dishes and top with fresh cilantro or parsley.
7. Serve.

Nutrition (per serving)

Calories: 220 Protein: 8g Carbohydrates: 34g Fat: 6g

Balsamic-Glazed Chicken with Greens

Prep Time: 10 minutes

Cook Time: 20 minutes

Servings: 4

Ingredients

- 4 boneless, skinless chicken breasts
- Salt and pepper, to taste
- 1 tbsp olive oil
- 1/4 cup of balsamic vinegar
- 1 tbsp honey (optional for added sweetness)
- 1 tsp Dijon mustard
- 1 tbsp olive oil
- 2 garlic cloves, minced
- 4 cups of fresh kale or Swiss chard, chopped (or a mix of both)
- Salt and pepper, to taste
- 1/4 cup of low-sodium chicken broth (or water)
- Lemon wedges, for garnish

Instructions

1. Season both sides of the chicken breasts with salt and pepper.
2. In a large pan, warm 1 tbsp olive oil over medium-high heat. Cook the chicken breasts on each side for 5-6 minutes until golden brown and well done. Remove the chicken from the skillet and put it aside.

3. Combine the balsamic vinegar, honey, and Dijon mustard in the same skillet. Stir thoroughly and let the mixture boil for 2-3 minutes or until slightly thickened. Return the chicken to the skillet and coat with the glaze. Remove from heat and cover to keep it warm.
4. In a separate pan, warm 1 tbsp olive oil over medium heat. Add the minced garlic and simmer for 1 minute, until fragrant. Season the chopped kale or Swiss chard with salt and pepper, then pour in the chicken broth. Sauté the greens for 3-4 minutes, stirring periodically, until wilted and tender.
5. Serve the balsamic-glazed chicken beside a large bowl of greens. Garnish with lemon wedges.

Nutrition (per serving)

Calories: 300 Protein: 32g Carbohydrates: 12g Fat: 12g Fiber: 3g

Cauliflower Rice Stir-Fry

Prep Time: 10 minutes Cook Time: 15 minutes Servings: 4

Ingredients

- 1 medium head of cauliflower, grated
- 1 tbsp coconut oil
- 1 small onion, finely chopped
- 1 red bell pepper, diced
- 1 cup of broccoli florets, chopped
- 1 medium carrot, julienned
- 1 zucchini, diced
- 2 garlic cloves, minced
- 1 tbsp ginger, minced
- 3 tbsp coconut aminos or low-sodium tamari
- 1/2 tsp turmeric powder
- 1/4 tsp black pepper
- 1/4 tsp sea salt (optional)
- Fresh cilantro, chopped, for garnish
- Lime wedges for serving

Instructions

1. Remove the cauliflower's leaves and core. Grate the cauliflower using a box grater or blend it in a food processor until it resembles rice. Set aside.

2. Heat the coconut oil over medium heat in a large skillet or wok. Sauté the onion, garlic, and ginger for 2–3 minutes, until aromatic.
3. Combine the bell pepper, broccoli, carrots, and zucchini. Stir-fry for 5-7 minutes until the veggies are soft and crisp.
4. Add the cauliflower rice to the skillet. Sprinkle with turmeric, black pepper, and optional sea salt. Stir well and simmer for 3-5 minutes or until the cauliflower rice is cooked.
5. Add the coconut aminos or tamari and mix to blend. Adjust the seasoning as required.
6. Garnish with fresh cilantro and lime juice. Serve warm.

Nutrition (per serving):

Calories: 110 kcal Carbohydrates: 14g Protein: 3g Fat: 5g Fiber: 5g Sugars: 5g

Sautéed Mushrooms with Garlic Kale

Prep Time: 5 minutes Cook Time: 15 minutes Servings: 2

Ingredients

- 1 tbsp olive oil or coconut oil
- 2 cups of mushrooms, sliced
- 3 cups of kale leaves, chopped
- 3 garlic cloves, minced
- 1/4 tsp sea salt
- 1/4 tsp black pepper
- 1 tsp lemon juice (optional for brightness)
- Fresh parsley, chopped, for garnish

Instructions

1. In a large skillet, heat the olive oil over medium heat. Cook the mushrooms for 5-7 minutes, until they are browned and softened.
2. Cook the garlic in the pan for 1-2 minutes, turning often to avoid browning.
3. Season the kale with sea salt and black pepper. Stir well and simmer for 3-5 minutes or until the kale is wilted and soft.
4. If preferred, add a sprinkle of lemon juice.
5. Garnish with chopped parsley and serve warm.

Nutrition (per serving):

Calories: 90 kcal Carbohydrates: 8g Protein: 3g Fat: 5g Fiber: 2g Sugars: 2g

Lemon Dill Salmon with Asparagus

Prep Time: 10 minutes

Cook Time: 15 minutes

Servings: 2

Ingredients

- 2 salmon fillets (about 6 ounces each)
- 1 tbsp olive oil, divided
- 1 tbsp fresh lemon juice
- 1 tsp lemon zest
- 1 tbsp fresh dill, chopped
- Salt and black pepper, to taste
- 1 bunch asparagus, trimmed
- Lemon wedges for serving

Instructions

1. Preheat the oven to 400 degrees Fahrenheit (200 degrees Celsius) and line a baking sheet with parchment paper.
2. Combine the lemon juice, zest, and dill in a small bowl. Set aside.
3. Place the salmon fillets on one side of the baking sheet. Drizzle half the olive oil over the fish and season with salt and pepper. Spread the lemon-dill mixture equally on each fillet.
4. Arrange the asparagus on the other side of the baking sheet. Drizzle with the remaining olive oil, then season with salt and pepper. Toss lightly to coat.
5. Bake for 12-15 minutes until the salmon is fully cooked and easily flaked with a fork and the asparagus is soft.
6. Serve with lemon wedges.

Nutrition (per serving):

Calories: 320 kcal Carbohydrates: 5g Protein: 30g Fat: 20g Fiber: 2g Sugars: 2g

Butternut Squash & Sage Risotto

Prep Time: 10 minutes

Cook Time: 30 minutes

Servings: 4

Ingredients

- 1 tbsp olive oil
- 1 small onion, finely chopped
- 2 garlic cloves, minced
- 1 cup of Arborio rice
- 1 cup of butternut squash, diced into small cubes
- 4 cups of low-sodium vegetable broth, warmed
- 1/4 cup of white wine (optional)
- 1 tbsp fresh sage, chopped
- 1/4 tsp sea salt
- 1/4 tsp black pepper
- 2 tbsp nutritional yeast
- Fresh parsley, chopped, for garnish

Instructions

1. Heat the olive oil over medium heat in a large skillet or saucepan. Sauté the onion and garlic for 3-4 minutes, until tender and aromatic.
2. Stir in the Arborio rice until fully coated with oil. Toast the rice for about 2 minutes, stirring continuously.
3. Add the butternut squash cubes and simmer for 2-3 minutes.
4. Pour in the white wine (if using) and simmer until almost absorbed.
5. Add the hot vegetable broth one ladle at a time, stirring constantly. Before adding the next broth, ensure the previous one has been absorbed. Continue cooking for 20-25 minutes or until the rice is creamy and soft.
6. Add the sage, salt, and black pepper when the risotto is almost done. If you want a cheese taste, add nutritional yeast.
7. Once the rice and squash are thoroughly cooked, remove from the heat and set aside for a minute. Garnish with fresh parsley and serve warm.

Nutrition (per serving):

Calories: 240 kcal Carbohydrates: 45g Protein: 5g Fat: 5g Fiber: 4g Sugars: 3g

Turmeric Chicken & Rice Pilaf

Prep Time: 10 minutes Cook Time: 30 minutes Servings: 4

Ingredients

- 2 tbsp olive oil or coconut oil divided
- 1 pound (450g) boneless, skinless chicken breast, diced
- 1 small onion, finely chopped
- 2 garlic cloves, minced
- 1 cup of basmati or jasmine rice, rinsed
- 1 1/2 cups of low-sodium chicken broth
- 1/2 cup of carrots, diced
- 1/2 cup of peas (fresh or frozen)
- 1 tsp ground turmeric
- 1/2 tsp ground cumin
- Salt and black pepper, to taste
- Fresh parsley or cilantro, chopped, for garnish

Instructions

1. Warm 1 tbsp olive oil over medium heat in a large skillet or saucepan. Add the diced chicken and season with salt and black pepper. Cook for 5–7 minutes or until the chicken is golden brown and cooked. Remove the chicken from the skillet and put it aside.
2. Heat the remaining olive oil in the same skillet and add the onion and garlic. Sauté the onion for 2-3 minutes until it is transparent and aromatic.
3. Combine the rice, carrots, and peas in the skillet, stirring to coat them with the oil and onion.
4. Stir in the turmeric and cumin, and simmer for another 1-2 minutes to let the spices unleash their flavors.
5. Pour in the chicken broth and mix well. Return the cooked chicken to the skillet and bring it to a simmer.
6. Cover the pan, lower the heat, and simmer for 15-18 minutes, or until the rice is cooked and the liquid has been absorbed.
7. Remove from the heat and allow the pilaf to resolve for 5 minutes before fluffing with a fork. Garnish with fresh cilantro or parsley and serve warm.

Nutrition (per serving):

Calories: 350 kcal Carbohydrates: 40g Protein: 22g Fat: 10g Fiber: 3g Sugars: 2g

Thai Coconut Curry Soup

Prep Time: 10 minutes Cook Time: 20 minutes Servings: 4

Ingredients

- 1 tbsp coconut oil
- 1 small onion, chopped
- 2 garlic cloves, minced
- 1 tbsp fresh ginger, grated
- 1 tbsp red curry paste
- 4 cups of low-sodium vegetable or chicken broth
- 1 can (14 ounces) full-fat coconut milk
- 1 medium sweet potato, peeled and diced
- 1 cup of carrots, sliced
- 1 cup of bell pepper, sliced (red or yellow)
- 1 cup of mushrooms, sliced
- 1 cup of baby spinach or kale leaves
- 1 tbsp fish sauce or tamari
- 1 tsp lime juice
- Fresh cilantro, chopped, for garnish
- Lime wedges for serving

Instructions

1. In a large saucepan, melt the coconut oil over medium heat. Sauté the onion, garlic, and ginger for 3-4 minutes, until aromatic and the onion softens.
2. Stir in the red curry paste and simmer for 1-2 minutes to unleash the flavors.
3. Pour in the vegetable or chicken broth and coconut milk, stirring until thoroughly combined. Bring the mixture to a moderate boil.
4. Put the sweet potato, carrots, and bell pepper into the saucepan. Reduce the heat to medium-low and cook for 10-12 minutes, until the veggies are soft.
5. Cook for another 3-5 minutes, until the mushrooms are tender and the greens have wilted.
6. Add the fish sauce or tamari, if using, and the lime juice. Adjust the seasoning as required.
7. Serve warm, topped with fresh cilantro and lime wedges on the side.

Nutrition (per serving):

Calories: 220 kcal Carbohydrates: 25g Protein: 4g Fat: 14g Fiber: 5g Sugars: 6g

Grilled Vegetable Paella

Prep Time: 15 minutes Cook Time: 35 minutes Servings: 4

Ingredients

- 2 tbsp olive oil, divided
- 1 cup of Arborio or short-grain rice
- 1 small onion, chopped
- 3 garlic cloves, minced
- 1 red bell pepper, sliced
- 1 yellow bell pepper, sliced
- 1 zucchini, sliced
- 1 cup of cherry tomatoes, halved
- 1 cup of green beans, trimmed
- 3 cups of low-sodium vegetable broth
- 1/2 tsp smoked paprika
- 1/4 tsp saffron threads, soaked in 2 tbsp warm water
- Salt and black pepper, to taste
- Fresh parsley, chopped, for garnish
- Lemon wedges for serving

Instructions

1. Preheat the grill or grill pan to medium-high heat. Toss the bell peppers, zucchini, cherry tomatoes, and green beans in 1 tbsp olive oil and season with salt and pepper.
2. Grill the veggies for 5-7 minutes, turning regularly, until lightly browned and tender. Set aside.
3. Heat the remaining 1 tbsp olive oil over medium heat in a large skillet or paella pan. Sauté the onion and garlic for 3-4 minutes, until softened.
4. Stir in the Arborio rice and simmer for 2-3 minutes to absorb the flavors.
5. Add the soaking water of the vegetable broth, smoked paprika, and saffron to the skillet. Bring to a low simmer and cook for 15-20 minutes, stirring periodically, until the rice is cooked and the liquid has been absorbed.
6. Add the grilled veggies to the rice and gently toss to incorporate. Adjust the salt and pepper to taste.
7. Remove from heat, add fresh parsley, and serve with lemon wedges on the side.

Nutrition (per serving):

Calories: 280 kcal Carbohydrates: 45g Protein: 6g Fat: 9g Fiber: 6g Sugars: 5g

Sweet Potato Shepherd's Pie

Prep Time: 15 minutes Cook Time: 35 minutes Servings: 4

Ingredients

- 2 large sweet potatoes, peeled and cubed
- 2 tbsp coconut milk (or almond milk)
- 1 tbsp olive oil
- Salt and black pepper, to taste
- 1 tbsp olive oil
- 1 small onion, chopped
- 2 garlic cloves, minced
- 1 medium carrot, diced
- 1 cup of mushrooms, chopped
- 1 cup of green peas (fresh or frozen)
- 1 cup of cooked lentils (or 1 can, drained and rinsed)
- 1/2 cup of vegetable broth
- 1 tbsp tomato paste
- 1 tsp fresh thyme (or 1/2 tsp dried)
- 1/2 tsp smoked paprika
- Salt and black pepper, to taste
- Fresh parsley, chopped, for garnish

Instructions

1. Preheat your oven to 400°F (200°C).
2. In a medium pot, boil the sweet potatoes until tender, about 10–12 minutes. Drain and return to the pot. Mash with coconut milk, olive oil, salt, and black pepper until smooth. Set aside.
3. While the potatoes cook, heat olive oil in a large skillet over medium heat. Add the onion and garlic and sauté for 3–4 minutes until softening.
4. Add the carrot, mushrooms, and green peas to the skillet. Cook for 5–7 minutes until the vegetables are tender.
5. Stir in the cooked lentils, vegetable broth, tomato paste, thyme, smoked paprika, salt, and black pepper. Simmer for 5 minutes, allowing the flavors to meld and the mixture to thicken slightly.
6. Spread the filling evenly in a baking dish. Spoon the mashed sweet potatoes over the top to cover the filling.
7. Bake in the oven for 15 minutes or until the top is lightly browned. Garnish with fresh parsley and serve warm.

Nutrition (per serving):

Calories: 320 kcal Carbohydrates: 50g Protein: 10g Fat: 9g Fiber: 10g Sugars: 10g

CHAPTER 4: SNACK RECIPES

Spicy Hummus and Veggie Platter

Prep Time: 10 minutes Cook Time: 0 minutes Servings: 4

Ingredients

- 1 can (15 ounces) chickpeas, drained and rinsed
- 2 tbsp tahini
- 2 tbsp olive oil
- 1 garlic clove, minced
- 1 tbsp lemon juice
- 1 tsp ground cumin
- 1/2 tsp smoked paprika
- 1/4 tsp cayenne pepper (adjust to your heat preference)
- Salt, to taste
- Water, as needed for desired consistency
- 1 cucumber, sliced into rounds
- 1 red bell pepper, sliced
- 1 small carrot, peeled and cut into sticks
- 1 cup of cherry tomatoes, halved
- 1 cup of celery sticks
- Fresh parsley or cilantro, chopped, for garnish

Instructions

1. Mix chickpeas, tahini, olive oil, garlic, lemon juice, cumin, smoked paprika, cayenne pepper, and salt in a food processor. Blend until smooth, adding water a little at a time to get the desired hummus consistency.
2. Season to taste; add lemon juice or cayenne for more flavor if desired.
3. Place the cucumber, bell pepper, carrot, cherry tomatoes, and celery sticks on a large serving plate.

4. Serve the spicy hummus in a small bowl in the middle of the plate, topped with fresh parsley or cilantro.
5. Enjoy.

Nutrition (per serving):

Calories: 180 kcal Carbohydrates: 20g Protein: 6g Fat: 9g Fiber: 6g Sugars: 6g

Cinnamon-Roasted Almonds

Prep Time: 5 minutes Cook Time: 15 minutes Servings: 4

Ingredients

- 1 1/2 cups of raw almonds
- 1 tbsp olive oil or coconut oil, melted
- 1 tbsp ground cinnamon
- 1 tbsp maple syrup or honey
- 1/4 tsp sea salt
- 1/4 tsp vanilla extract (optional)

Instructions

1. Preheat the oven to 350°F/175°C and line a baking sheet with parchment paper.
2. In a mixing bowl, combine the almonds, olive or coconut oil, cinnamon, maple syrup (if used), sea salt, and vanilla extract until equally coated.
3. Spread the almonds out in a single layer on the prepared baking sheet.
4. Roast the almonds in a preheated oven for 12-15 minutes, stirring halfway through, until golden brown and aromatic.
5. Remove from the oven and let to cool fully on the baking sheet.
6. Keep in an airtight jar for up to one week. Enjoy.

Nutrition (per serving):

Calories: 160 kcal Carbohydrates: 7g Protein: 6g Fat: 14g Fiber: 3g Sugars: 2g

Coconut Energy Bites

Prep Time: 10 minutes

Cook Time: 0 minutes

Servings: 12 bites

Ingredients

- 1 cup of unsweetened shredded coconut
- 1/2 cup of rolled oats
- 1/4 cup of almond butter (or other nut butter)
- 2 tbsp honey or maple syrup
- 1 tbsp chia seeds (optional)
- 1 tsp vanilla extract
- 1/4 tsp ground cinnamon
- Pinch of sea salt

Instructions

1. Combine the shredded coconut, oats, almond butter, honey (or maple syrup), chia seeds (optional), vanilla extract, cinnamon, and sea salt in a large mixing bowl.
2. Mix everything until fully blended. The mixture should feel somewhat sticky.
3. Roll the mixture into 12 tiny balls approximately an inch in diameter.
4. Place the energy bites on a baking sheet or dish with parchment paper.
5. Refrigerate for at least 30 minutes until firm.
6. Refrigerate in an airtight jar for up to a week.
7. Enjoy.

Nutrition (per serving):

Calories: 140 kcal Carbohydrates: 14g Protein: 4g Fat: 9g Fiber: 3g Sugars: 6g

Green Apple with Almond Butter

Prep Time: 5 minutes

Cook Time: 0 minutes

Servings: 1

Ingredients

- 1 medium green apple cored and sliced
- 2 tbsp almond butter
- A sprinkle of cinnamon (optional)
- A few crushed almonds or seeds

Instructions

1. Core and cut the green apple into wedges.
2. Place the almond butter in a small bowl or apply it straight over the apple slices.
3. For extra taste, sprinkle with cinnamon.
4. For an additional crunch, sprinkle with crushed almonds or seeds.
5. Enjoy right now.

Nutrition (per serving):

Calories: 180 kcal Carbohydrates: 22g Protein: 4g Fat: 10g Fiber: 5g Sugars: 15g

Roasted Chickpeas with Herbs

Prep Time: 10 minutes

Cook Time: 30 minutes

Servings: 4

Ingredients

- 1 can (15 ounces) chickpeas, drained and rinsed
- 1 tbsp olive oil
- 1 tsp dried rosemary
- 1 tsp dried thyme
- 1/2 tsp garlic powder
- 1/2 tsp smoked paprika
- 1/4 tsp sea salt
- 1/4 tsp black pepper
- Fresh lemon zest (optional, for garnish)

Instructions

1. Preheat the oven to 400 degrees Fahrenheit (200 degrees Celsius) and line a baking sheet with parchment paper.
2. Pat the chickpeas dry with a paper towel to remove any extra moisture.
3. Toss the chickpeas in a bowl with olive oil, rosemary, thyme, garlic powder, smoked paprika, sea salt, and black pepper until well combined.
4. Place the chickpeas in a single layer on the prepared baking sheet.
5. Roast the chickpeas in a preheated oven for 25-30 minutes, stirring halfway through, until golden and crispy.
6. Allow the chickpeas to cool for a few minutes before serving with a sprinkling of fresh lemon zest if preferred.
7. Serve and Enjoy.

Nutrition (per serving):

Calories: 120 kcal Carbohydrates: 18g Protein: 6g Fat: 4g Fiber: 5g Sugars: 1g

Turmeric-Spiced Trail Mix

Prep Time: 10 minutes

Cook Time: 0 minutes

Servings: 4

Ingredients

- 1/2 cup of raw almonds
- 1/2 cup of raw cashews
- 1/4 cup of pumpkin seeds (pepitas)
- 1/4 cup of sunflower seeds
- 1/4 cup of dried unsweetened cranberries or raisins
- 1/4 tsp ground turmeric
- 1/4 tsp ground cinnamon
- 1/4 tsp black pepper (to enhance turmeric absorption)
- 1 tbsp olive oil or coconut oil, melted
- 1/2 tsp sea salt (optional)

Instructions

1. Add almonds, cashews, pumpkin seeds, sunflower seeds, and dried cranberries or raisins in a large mixing bowl.
2. In a small mixing bowl, blend the turmeric, cinnamon, black pepper, and melted oil until well combined.
3. Drizzle the turmeric-spice mixture over the nuts and seeds and toss to coat.
4. If desired, season with a pinch of sea salt and combine again.
5. Keep in an airtight jar for up to one week.
6. Enjoy.

Nutrition (per serving):

Calories: 180 kcal Carbohydrates: 12g Protein: 6g Fat: 14g Fiber: 3g Sugars: 5g

Coconut Yogurt & Berry Dip

Prep Time: 5 minutes

Cook Time: 0 minutes

Servings: 4

Ingredients

- 1 cup of coconut yogurt (unsweetened)
- 1 tbsp honey or maple syrup
- 1 tsp vanilla extract
- 1/2 tsp ground cinnamon (optional)
- 1 cup of mixed berries
- Fresh mint leaves, for garnish (optional)

Instructions

1. Mix the coconut yogurt, honey (or maple syrup), vanilla extract, and cinnamon in a bowl. Stir until smooth and well combined.
2. Transfer the yogurt mixture to a serving bowl.
3. Arrange the fresh mixed berries around the dip to facilitate dipping.
4. Garnish with fresh mint leaves if preferred.
5. Serve immediately.

Nutrition (per serving):

Calories: 120 kcal Carbohydrates: 18g Protein: 2g Fat: 6g Fiber: 4g Sugars: 12g

Dark Chocolate Almond Bark

Prep Time: 10 minutes

Cook Time: 10 minutes

Servings: 4

Ingredients

- 1 cup of dark chocolate
- 1/2 cup of raw almonds, roughly chopped
- 1 tbsp chia seeds (optional)
- 1/2 tsp sea salt
- 1 tsp vanilla extract (optional)

Instructions

1. Line a baking sheet with parchment paper or a silicone baking mat.
2. In a heatproof bowl, melt the dark chocolate. You may do this by microwaving the chocolate in 30-second intervals and stirring between each or by using a double boiler.
3. Once melted, add the vanilla extract (if using) and pour the chocolate over the prepared baking sheet. Spread it evenly, approximately 1/4 inch thick.
4. Sprinkle the chopped almonds, chia seeds (if using), and sea salt over the melted chocolate.
5. Put the baking sheet in the refrigerator for approximately 30 minutes or until the chocolate is set and solid.
6. Once firm, split the bark into pieces and serve right away.

Nutrition (per serving):

Calories: 180 kcal Carbohydrates: 12g Protein: 4g Fat: 14g Fiber: 3g Sugars: 6g

Cashew Energy Bars

Prep Time: 10 minutes

Cook Time: 10 minutes

Servings: 8 bars

Ingredients

- 1 cup of raw cashews
- 1/2 cup of rolled oats
- 1/4 cup of unsweetened shredded coconut
- 2 tbsp chia seeds
- 2 tbsp almond butter (or any nut butter)
- 1/4 cup of honey or maple syrup
- 1 tsp vanilla extract
- Pinch of sea salt

Instructions

1. Put the cashews, oats, shredded coconut, chia seeds, and sea salt in a food processor. Pulse until the cashews are broken into tiny bits but not fully ground.
2. In a small mixing bowl, combine the almond butter, honey (or maple syrup), and vanilla extract until smooth.
3. Add the wet ingredients to the food processor and pulse until well blended, and the mixture holds together when squeezed.
4. Line a small (8x8-inch) baking dish with parchment paper. Press the mixture evenly into the bowl.
5. Refrigerate for 30 minutes to enable the bars to firm up.
6. Once cold, cut into 8 bars and refrigerate in an airtight jar for up to a week.

Nutrition (per serving):

Calories: 180 kcal Carbohydrates: 15g Protein: 5g Fat: 12g Fiber: 3g Sugars: 7g

Cucumber & Avocado Salsa

Prep Time: 10 minutes

Cook Time: 0 minutes

Servings: 4

Ingredients

- 1 large cucumber, diced
- 1 ripe avocado, diced
- 1 small red onion, finely chopped
- 1/2 cup of cherry tomatoes, halved
- 1 tbsp fresh lime juice
- 1 tbsp olive oil
- 1 tbsp fresh cilantro, chopped
- Salt and black pepper, to taste

Instructions

1. Add the chopped cucumber, avocado, red onion, and cherry tomatoes to a medium mixing bowl.
2. Drizzle the mixture with lime juice and olive oil, then gently toss to incorporate.
3. Sprinkle with fresh cilantro and season with salt and black pepper to taste.
4. Serve immediately.

Nutrition (per serving):

Calories: 120 kcal Carbohydrates: 10g Protein: 2g Fat: 9g Fiber: 6g Sugars: 4g

Almond Butter & Date Stuffed Apples

Prep Time: 10 minutes

Cook Time: 20 minutes

Servings: 4

Ingredients

- 4 medium apples
- 1/4 cup of almond butter
- 6 pitted dates, chopped
- 1/4 tsp cinnamon
- 1 tbsp chopped walnuts or pecans (optional)
- 1 tbsp honey (optional)
- 1/2 tsp vanilla extract (optional)

Instructions

1. Preheat the oven to 350°F (175° C). Slice off the tops of the apples and scoop out the cores, leaving a hollow hole in the middle of each. Take caution not to cut through the bottom.
2. Combine the almond butter, sliced dates, cinnamon, optional honey, and vanilla extract in a small mixing bowl.
3. Fill each apple with the almond butter and date mixture, gently pushing down to compress it.
4. Place the packed apples in a baking dish and loosely wrap them with foil.
5. Bake for 20 minutes until the apples are soft, and the filling is heated.
6. To add crunch, sprinkle chopped walnuts or pecans on top of each filled apple.
7. Serve warm.

Nutrition (per serving):

Calories: 210 kcal Carbohydrates: 30g Protein: 4g Fat: 9g Fiber: 6g Sugars: 20g

Baked Kale Chips with Sea Salt

Prep Time: 10 minutes

Cook Time: 15 minutes

Servings: 4

Ingredients

- 1 bunch kale, washed and dried
- 1 tbsp olive oil
- 1/2 tsp sea salt (or to taste)
- 1/4 tsp black pepper (optional)
- 1/4 tsp garlic powder (optional)

Instructions

1. Preheat the oven to 350°F/175°C and line a baking sheet with parchment paper.
2. Remove the kale stems and shred the leaves into bite-size pieces. To avoid soggy chips, ensure that the kale has been well-dried.
3. Combine the kale, olive oil, sea salt, and other spices (black pepper and garlic powder) in a large mixing bowl.
4. Spread the kale in a single layer on the baking sheet, ensuring the leaves aren't crowded.
5. Bake for 10-15 minutes, until the kale is crispy and the edges are gently browned. Kale chips may burn rapidly, so check them constantly.
6. Remove from the oven and let to cool on the baking sheet. Serve immediately and enjoy.

Nutrition (per serving):

Calories: 60 kcal Carbohydrates: 10g Protein: 2g Fat: 3g Fiber: 2g Sugars: 1g

Carrot & Ginger Dip with Veggies

Prep Time: 10 minutes

Cook Time: 0 minutes

Servings: 4

Ingredients

- 2 large carrots, peeled and chopped
- 1 tbsp fresh ginger, grated
- 1/4 cup of tahini (or almond butter)
- 2 tbsp fresh lemon juice
- 1 tbsp olive oil
- 1/2 tsp ground cumin
- 1/4 tsp sea salt
- 1/4 tsp black pepper
- Water, as needed for desired consistency
- Fresh veggies (cucumber, bell peppers, celery, and cherry tomatoes) for dipping

Instructions

1. Add carrots, grated ginger, tahini, lemon juice, olive oil, cumin, salt, and black pepper in a food processor or blender.
2. Blend until smooth, adding water a little at a time to get the desired dip consistency.
3. Taste and adjust the seasoning, adding more salt, pepper, or lemon juice as required.
4. Serve the carrot and ginger dip with fresh vegetables, such as cucumber, bell peppers, celery, and cherry tomatoes.

Nutrition (per serving):

Calories: 120 kcal Carbohydrates: 18g Protein: 3g Fat: 6g Fiber: 5g Sugars: 7g

Spiced Pumpkin Seed Clusters

Prep Time: 10 minutes

Cook Time: 15 minutes

Servings: 4

Ingredients

- 1 cup of raw pumpkin seeds (pepitas)
- 1 tbsp olive oil or coconut oil
- 1 tsp ground cinnamon
- 1/2 tsp ground ginger
- 1/4 tsp ground nutmeg
- 1/4 tsp cayenne pepper (optional, for a spicy kick)
- 1 tbsp maple syrup or honey
- 1/4 tsp sea salt
- 1 tsp vanilla extract (optional)

Instructions

1. Preheat the oven to 350°F/175°C and line a baking sheet with parchment paper.
2. Add the pumpkin seeds, olive oil, cinnamon, ginger, nutmeg, cayenne pepper (if desired), maple syrup (or honey), and sea salt in a large mixing bowl. Stir the seeds until they are uniformly covered.
3. Place the pumpkin seeds in a single layer on the prepared baking sheet.
4. Bake for 10-15 minutes, stirring halfway through, until the seeds become brown and aromatic. Pay special attention to prevent burning.
5. Remove from the oven and let the clusters to cool fully. Once cold, separate the seeds into clusters.
6. Keep in an airtight jar at room temperature for up to a week.

Nutrition (per serving):

Calories: 150 kcal Carbohydrates: 12g Protein: 6g Fat: 10g Fiber: 3g Sugars: 4g

Chia Seed Crackers with Hummus

Prep Time: 10 minutes

Cook Time: 25 minutes

Servings: 4

Ingredients

- 1/2 cup of chia seeds
- 1/2 cup of water
- 1/2 cup of almond flour or coconut flour
- 1 tbsp olive oil
- 1/2 tsp sea salt
- 1/4 tsp garlic powder (optional)
- 1/4 tsp onion powder (optional)
- 1 cup of homemade or store-bought hummus (preferably low-sodium and plain)

Instructions

1. Preheat the oven to 350°F/175°C and line a baking sheet with parchment paper.
2. In a small bowl, mix the chia seeds and water. Allow it to rest for approximately 5 minutes so the chia seeds absorb the water and produce a gel-like consistency.
3. Combine the almond flour (or coconut flour), olive oil, sea salt, and optional garlic and onion powder into the chia mixture. Stir until entirely blended, creating a dough-like consistency.
4. Roll out the dough between two pieces of parchment paper to a thickness of approximately 1/8 inch.
5. Remove the top layer of parchment paper and divide the dough into cracker-sized squares or rectangles.
6. Place the dough on the prepared baking sheet and bake for 20-25 minutes or until golden and crisp. Allow them to cool fully on the baking pan.
7. Serve cooled chia seed crackers with hummus on the side for dipping.

Nutrition (per serving):

Calories: 160 kcal Carbohydrates: 10g Protein: 5g Fat: 12g Fiber: 7g Sugars: 1g

Zesty Lemon Energy Balls

Prep Time: 10 minutes

Cook Time: 0 minutes

Servings: 12 balls

Ingredients

- 1 cup of rolled oats
- 1/2 cup of almond meal or cashew flour
- 1/4 cup of unsweetened shredded coconut
- 1/4 cup of almond butter (or any nut butter)
- 2 tbsp honey or maple syrup
- Zest of 1 lemon
- 2 tbsp fresh lemon juice
- 1/4 tsp vanilla extract
- 1 tbsp chia seeds (optional)
- Pinch of sea salt

Instructions

1. In a medium bowl, mix the rolled oats, almond meal, shredded coconut, almond butter, honey (or maple syrup), lemon zest, lemon juice, vanilla extract, chia seeds (if using), and sea salt.
2. Stir everything up until well blended. The mixture should be somewhat sticky and easily formed into balls.
3. Roll the mixture into 12 small balls approximately an inch in diameter.
4. Place the energy balls on a parchment-lined baking sheet or dish.
5. Refrigerate for at least 30 minutes until firm.
6. Refrigerate in an airtight jar for up to a week. Enjoy.

Nutrition (per serving):

Calories: 140 kcal Carbohydrates: 15g Protein: 4g Fat: 9g Fiber: 3g Sugars: 8g

Avocado-Cucumber Slices with Sea Salt

Prep Time: 5 minutes

Cook Time: 0 minutes

Servings: 2

Ingredients

- 1 large cucumber, sliced into rounds
- 1 ripe avocado, peeled and sliced
- 1/4 tsp sea salt (or to taste)
- 1/4 tsp black pepper (optional)
- 1 tbsp fresh lemon juice (optional)
- Fresh dill or parsley, chopped, for garnish (optional)

Instructions

1. Slice the cucumber into rounds and the avocado into thin slices.
2. Arrange the cucumber slices on a platter, then carefully arrange the avocado slices on top.
3. To season, sprinkle with sea salt and black pepper (if using).
4. Drizzle with fresh lemon juice and sprinkle with chopped dill or parsley for added taste and freshness.
5. Serve immediately.

Nutrition (per serving):

Calories: 160 kcal Carbohydrates: 12g Protein: 2g Fat: 14g Fiber: 7g Sugars: 4g

Dark Chocolate Avocado Mousse

Prep Time: 10 minutes

Cook Time: 0 minutes

Servings: 4

Ingredients

- 2 ripe avocados, peeled and pitted
- 1/4 cup of unsweetened cocoa powder
- 1/4 cup of maple syrup or honey (adjust to taste)
- 1 tsp vanilla extract
- 1/4 cup of almond milk or coconut milk
- Pinch of sea salt
- 2 tbsp dark chocolate chips
- Fresh berries, for garnish (optional)

Instructions

1. Add ripe avocados, chocolate powder, maple syrup (or honey), vanilla extract, almond milk, and sea salt in a blender or food processor.
2. Blend until smooth and creamy. If the mousse is too thick, add almond milk gradually until it reaches the appropriate consistency.
3. Taste and adjust the sweetness, adding more maple syrup or honey as needed.
4. Spoon the mousse into separate serving plates and chill for at least 30 minutes.
5. Before serving, top with fresh berries and optional dark chocolate chips.

Nutrition (per serving):

Calories: 180 kcal Carbohydrates: 16g Protein: 3g Fat: 12g Fiber: 6g Sugars: 9g

Coconut & Berry Chia Pudding

Prep Time: 5 minutes

Cook Time: 0 minutes

Servings: 2

Ingredients

- 1/2 cup of chia seeds
- 1 cup of coconut milk (unsweetened)
- 1 tbsp maple syrup or honey
- 1/2 tsp vanilla extract
- 1/4 cup of mixed berries
- 1 tbsp shredded unsweetened coconut (optional, for garnish)
- Fresh mint leaves (optional, for garnish)

Instructions

1. Blend the chia seeds, coconut milk, maple syrup (or honey), and vanilla extract in a bowl or jar. Stir thoroughly to ensure the chia seeds are uniformly dispersed.
2. Cover the bowl or jar and chill for at least 2 hours, preferably overnight, to let the chia seeds absorb the liquid and thicken into a pudding-like consistency.
3. When the pudding is done, please stir it thoroughly and divide it into two serving bowls or glasses.
4. Top with fresh mixed berries, shredded coconut, and fresh mint leaves for garnish.
5. Serve chilled, and enjoy.

Nutrition (per serving):

Calories: 180 kcal Carbohydrates: 20g Protein: 4g Fat: 10g Fiber: 9g Sugars: 6g

Almond Flour Banana Bread

Prep Time: 10 minutes Cook Time: 45 minutes Servings: 8

Ingredients

- 2 ripe bananas, mashed
- 2 cups of almond flour
- 3 large eggs
- 1/4 cup of honey or maple syrup
- 1/4 cup of coconut oil, melted (or butter)
- 1 tsp vanilla extract
- 1 tsp baking powder
- 1/2 tsp ground cinnamon
- 1/4 tsp sea salt
- 1/4 tsp baking soda
- Optional: 1/2 cup of chopped walnuts or dark chocolate chips (for added texture)

Instructions

1. Preheat the oven to 350°F (175° C). Grease the loaf pan or line it with parchment paper.
2. Mash the ripe bananas using a fork or potato masher in a large mixing bowl until smooth.
3. Mix the eggs, honey (or maple syrup), melted coconut oil (or butter), and vanilla extract into the mashed bananas. Mix until well mixed.
4. Combine almond flour, baking powder, baking soda, cinnamon, and sea salt in a separate bowl.
5. Gradually mix the dry and wet ingredients, stirring until just blended. If using, mix in the chopped walnuts or dark chocolate chips.
6. Pour the batter into the prepared loaf pan and use a spatula to smooth the top.
7. Bake for 40 to 45 minutes or until a toothpick inserted in the middle comes out clean.
8. Allow the bread to cool for 10 minutes in the pan before transferring it to a wire rack to finish cooling before slicing.

Nutrition (per serving):

Calories: 180 kcal Carbohydrates: 15g Protein: 7g Fat: 14g Fiber: 4g Sugars: 9g

Baked Apple with Cinnamon

Prep Time: 5 minutes

Cook Time: 25 minutes

Servings: 2

Ingredients

- 2 medium apples
- 1 tbsp cinnamon
- 1 tbsp maple syrup or honey (
- 1/4 tsp ground nutmeg (optional)
- 1 tbsp chopped walnuts or almonds (optional, for crunch)
- 1/2 tsp vanilla extract (optional)

Instructions

1. Preheat the oven to 350°F (175° C).
2. Core the apples while keeping the bottoms intact to form a hollow core for filling.
3. Combine the cinnamon, nutmeg (if using), and maple syrup or honey in a small bowl.
4. Spoon the cinnamon mixture into the apples' hollow centers, pushing down slightly to compact it.
5. Put the apples in a baking dish. Put chopped walnuts or almonds on top of the apples for desired texture.
6. Bake the apples for 20-25 minutes or until soft and the cinnamon filling bubbles.
7. Remove from the oven and let to cool slightly before serving.

Nutrition (per serving):

Calories: 150 kcal Carbohydrates: 35g Protein: 1g Fat: 1g Fiber: 5g Sugars: 30g

Choco-Coconut Energy Balls

Prep Time: 10 minutes

Cook Time: 0 minutes

Servings: 12

Ingredients

- 1 cup of unsweetened shredded coconut
- 1/2 cup of almond butter (or any nut butter)
- 1/4 cup of cocoa powder (unsweetened)
- 1/4 cup of honey or maple syrup
- 1/2 tsp vanilla extract
- 1/4 cup of dark chocolate chips (optional)
- Pinch of sea salt
- 2 tbsp chia seeds or flaxseeds (optional)

Instructions

1. Mix the shredded coconut, almond butter, cocoa powder, honey (or maple syrup), vanilla extract, and a sprinkle of sea salt in a medium bowl. Stir until everything is fully combined.
2. Add the chia seeds or flaxseeds and blend well if you want more texture.
3. Fold in the dark chocolate chips for a deeper taste.
4. Roll the mixture into little balls approximately an inch in diameter. You should have roughly 12 balls.
5. Place the energy balls on a parchment-lined baking sheet or dish.
6. Refrigerate for at least 30 minutes until firm.
7. Refrigerate in an airtight jar for up to a week.

Nutrition (per serving):

Calories: 150 kcal Carbohydrates: 12g Protein: 4g Fat: 10g Fiber: 4g Sugars: 8g

Matcha Coconut Bliss Bites

Prep Time: 10 minutes

Cook Time: 0 minutes

Servings: 12 bites

Ingredients

- 1 cup of unsweetened shredded coconut
- 1/2 cup of almond flour (or coconut flour)
- 2 tbsp coconut oil, melted
- 2 tbsp maple syrup or honey
- 1 tbsp matcha powder
- 1/4 tsp vanilla extract
- Pinch of sea salt

Instructions

1. Mix the shredded coconut, almond flour, matcha powder, and sea salt in a mixing bowl.
2. Combine the melted coconut oil, maple syrup (or honey), and vanilla extract. Stir until everything is well combined and the mixture starts to cling together.
3. Roll the mixture into little 1-inch balls with your hands.
4. Place the bits on a parchment-lined tray and chill to harden for at least 30 minutes.
5. Once cooled, serve and enjoy.

Nutrition (per serving):

Calories: 160 kcal Carbohydrates: 10g Protein: 3g Fat: 14g Fiber: 5g Sugars: 5g

Roasted Pears with Walnuts

Prep Time: 10 minutes

Cook Time: 25 minutes

Servings: 4

Ingredients

- 4 ripe pears, halved and cored
- 1 tbsp olive oil or melted coconut oil
- 1/4 tsp ground cinnamon
- 1/4 tsp ground nutmeg (optional)
- 1/4 cup of walnuts, roughly chopped
- 1 tbsp honey or maple syrup (optional for sweetness)
- 1 tbsp fresh lemon juice
- Fresh mint leaves, for garnish (optional)

Instructions

1. Preheat the oven to 375°F (190°C), and line a baking sheet with parchment paper.
2. Cut the pears in half and take off the cores. Place the pears cut side up on the prepared baking sheet.
3. Drizzle the pears with olive oil (or melted coconut oil) and season with cinnamon and nutmeg (if desired).
4. Roast the pears in a warm oven for 20-25 minutes or until soft and gently browned.
5. While the pears roast, toast the chopped walnuts in a dry pan over medium heat for 3-4 minutes, turning periodically until aromatic and lightly browned.
6. When the pears are done, sprinkle with honey or maple syrup, then squeeze fresh lemon juice on top.
7. Sprinkle the roasted walnuts over the pears and garnish with fresh mint leaves, if preferred.
8. Serve warm and enjoy.

Nutrition (per serving):

Calories: 180 kcal Carbohydrates: 30g Protein: 3g Fat: 8g Fiber: 5g Sugars: 20g

Cashew Cream Fruit Tart

Prep Time: 15 minutes

Cook Time: 0 minutes

Servings: 6

Ingredients

- 1 cup of almond flour
- 1/2 cup of unsweetened shredded coconut
- 2 tbsp coconut oil, melted
- 2 tbsp maple syrup or honey
- Pinch of sea salt
- 1 cup of raw cashews, soaked for 4 hours or overnight
- 1/4 cup of coconut milk (or almond milk)
- 2 tbsp maple syrup or honey
- 1 tsp vanilla extract
- Pinch of sea salt
- 1 cup of mixed fresh berries
- 1 tbsp shredded coconut (optional, for garnish)

Instructions

1. Add almond flour, shredded coconut, melted coconut oil, maple syrup (or honey), and sea salt in a mixing bowl. Stir until the ingredients come together into a dough.
2. Press the crust mixture into the bottom of a tart pan, making an equal layer. Press hard to form a tight crust.
3. Refrigerate the crust while you make the cashew cream filling.
4. Drain the soaked cashews and transfer them to a high-speed blender or food processor. Combine coconut milk, maple syrup (or honey), vanilla extract, and sea salt. Blend until smooth and creamy, scraping down the sides as necessary. If the mixture is too thick, add more coconut milk until you get the ideal consistency.
5. Spread the cashew cream filling evenly on the cold crust. Smooth the top using a spatula.
6. Place the mixed berries on top of the cashew cream. Sprinkle with shredded coconut for extra texture.
7. Refrigerate the tart for at least 2 hours before serving so that it may thicken up and cold.
8. Slice and serve.

Nutrition (per serving):

Calories: 250 kcal Carbohydrates: 20g Protein: 5g Fat: 18g Fiber: 4g Sugars: 12g

Avocado Cacao Pudding

Prep Time: 5 minutes Cook Time: 0 minutes Servings: 4

Ingredients

- 2 ripe avocados, peeled and pitted
- 1/4 cup of unsweetened cocoa powder
- 2–3 tbsp maple syrup or honey (to taste)
- 1 tsp vanilla extract
- 1/4 cup of almond milk
- Pinch of sea salt
- Optional toppings: fresh berries, shredded coconut, or a sprinkle of cacao nibs

Instructions

1. Add ripe avocados, chocolate powder, maple syrup (or honey), vanilla extract, almond milk, and sea salt in a blender or food processor.
2. Blend until smooth and creamy, scraping down the sides to ensure everything is well blended.
3. Adjust the pudding's sweetness by adding more maple syrup or honey, if desired.
4. Divide the pudding amongst separate serving bowls or glasses.
5. Refrigerate for 30 minutes to enable the pudding to firm up.
6. Sprinkle over fresh berries, shredded coconut, or cacao nibs for extra texture and taste.
7. Serve cold, and enjoy.

Nutrition (per serving):

Calories: 180 kcal Carbohydrates: 18g Protein: 3g Fat: 12g Fiber: 7g Sugars: 10g

Mango Coconut Sorbet

Prep Time: 10 minutes

Freezing Time: 4 hours

Servings: 4

Ingredients

- 2 ripe mangoes, peeled and chopped
- 1/2 cup of coconut milk (unsweetened)
- 1 tbsp honey or maple syrup
- 1 tbsp fresh lime juice
- Pinch of sea salt

Instructions

1. Combine the diced mangos, coconut milk, honey lime juice, and a sprinkle of sea salt in a blender or food processor.
2. Blend until smooth and creamy, scraping down the sides as necessary.
3. Pour the mango mixture into a shallow jar and distribute evenly.
4. Freeze for at least four hours or until firm.
5. To get a light, fluffy texture, scrape and fluff the sorbet after it has been frozen.
6. Serve in bowls or glasses and enjoy.

Nutrition (per serving):

Calories: 140 kcal Carbohydrates: 36g Protein: 1g Fat: 4g Fiber: 3g Sugars: 30g

Lemon Blueberry Almond Cake

Prep Time: 15 minutes Cook Time: 30 minutes Servings: 8

Ingredients

- 2 cups of almond flour
- 1/4 cup of coconut flour
- 1 tsp baking powder
- 1/2 tsp baking soda
- 1/4 tsp sea salt
- 3 large eggs
- 1/4 cup of maple syrup or honey
- 1/4 cup of coconut oil, melted
- 1/4 cup of unsweetened almond milk (or other plant-based milk)
- Zest of 1 lemon
- 2 tbsp fresh lemon juice
- 1 tsp vanilla extract
- 1 cup of fresh blueberries (or frozen, thawed)

Instructions

1. Preheat the oven to 350°F (175°C). Grease or line an 8-inch round cake pan with parchment paper.
2. Add almond flour, coconut flour, baking powder, baking soda, and sea salt in a large mixing bowl.
3. Combine the eggs, maple syrup (or honey), melted coconut oil, almond milk, lemon zest, lemon juice, and vanilla extract in a separate mixing bowl.
4. Pour the wet ingredients into the dry ingredients and stir just until mixed.
5. Gently fold in the blueberries until equally distributed throughout the batter.
6. Pour the batter into the prepared cake pan and spread evenly.
7. Bake for 25-30 minutes, or until a toothpick inserted in the middle comes out clean and the top is gently browned.
8. Let the cake sit in the pan for 10 minutes before cooling it to a wire rack.
9. Serve and enjoy.

Nutrition (per serving):

Calories: 220 kcal Carbohydrates: 18g Protein: 6g Fat: 16g Fiber: 6g Sugars: 10g

Cinnamon-Spiced Baked Apples

Prep Time: 10 minutes

Cook Time: 25 minutes

Servings: 4

Ingredients

- 4 medium apples (such as Gala or Fuji), cored
- 1/4 cup of raisins or chopped dates
- 1/4 cup of chopped walnuts or pecans (optional)
- 1 tsp ground cinnamon
- 1/4 tsp ground nutmeg (optional)
- 2 tbsp maple syrup or honey
- 1/4 cup of water
- 1/2 tsp vanilla extract (optional)

Instructions

1. Preheat the oven to 350°F/175°C and gently butter a baking dish.
2. Core the apples, keeping the bottoms intact to contain the filling. You may use either an apple corer or a little knife.
3. Combine raisins or chopped dates, walnuts (if using), cinnamon, and nutmeg in a small mixing bowl.
4. Stuff the mixture into the cored apples, carefully pushing to fill the centers.
5. Put the apples in the prepared baking dish. Drizzle maple syrup (or honey) and vanilla extract (if used) on each apple.
6. Pour water into the bottom of the baking dish to keep the apples wet during baking.
7. Bake the apples for 25–30 minutes until soft and golden brown. Baste the apples with the liquid in the baking dish halfway through.
8. Allow the apples to cool slightly before serving. Serve warm.

Nutrition (per serving):

Calories: 180 kcal Carbohydrates: 46g Protein: 2g Fat: 3g Fiber: 6g Sugars: 30g

Vanilla Chia Pudding with Berries

Prep Time: 5 minutes

Chill Time: 2 hours

Servings: 2

Ingredients

- 1/2 cup of chia seeds
- 1 cup of unsweetened almond milk
- 1 tbsp maple syrup or honey
- 1 tsp vanilla extract
- Pinch of sea salt
- 1/2 cup of mixed fresh berries
- 1 tbsp shredded coconut (optional, for garnish)

Instructions

1. Combine the almond milk, chia seeds, maple syrup (or honey), vanilla extract, and sea salt in a mixing bowl or jar. Stir well to ensure that the chia seeds are uniformly dispersed.
2. Cover and chill the mixture for at least 2 hours, preferably overnight, to let the chia seeds absorb the liquid and thicken into a pudding-like consistency.
3. Once the pudding has thickened, give it a vigorous stir. If the pudding is too thick, add more almond milk until you get the required consistency.
4. Divide the pudding into two serving bowls or glasses.
5. Garnish with fresh mixed berries and, if wanted, shredded coconut.
6. Serve chilled to enjoy.

Nutrition (per serving):

Calories: 150 kcal Carbohydrates: 20g Protein: 5g Fat: 7g Fiber: 10g Sugars: 8g

Cocoa-Almond Protein Bites

Prep Time: 10 minutes

Chill Time: 30 minutes

Servings: 12

Ingredients

- 1 cup of raw almonds
- 1/4 cup of unsweetened cocoa powder
- 1/4 cup of protein powder (preferably plant-based)
- 2 tbsp almond butter (or any nut butter)
- 2 tbsp honey or maple syrup
- 1 tbsp chia seeds or flaxseeds (optional)
- 1/4 tsp vanilla extract
- 1/4 tsp sea salt
- 2 tbsp water (more if needed to bind the mixture)

Instructions

1. In a food processor, pulse the almonds until finely chopped but not ground (texture is important).
2. Combine the cocoa powder, protein powder, almond butter, honey (or maple syrup), chia seeds (if using), vanilla extract, and sea salt in a food processor. Pulse the mixture until it begins to come together.
3. Add water one tbsp at a time until the dough-like substance is easily pushed together with your palms.
4. Roll the mixture into little balls approximately an inch in diameter. You should receive around 12 protein bits.
5. Place the bits on a parchment-lined tray and chill to harden for at least 30 minutes.
6. Refrigerate in an airtight jar for up to a week. Enjoy.

Nutrition (per serving):

Calories: 160 kcal Carbohydrates: 10g Protein: 8g Fat: 12g Fiber: 3g Sugars: 6g

Pumpkin Spice Coconut Custard

Prep Time: 10 minutes

Cook Time: 30 minutes

Servings: 4

Ingredients

- 1 can (14 ounces) full-fat coconut milk
- 1/2 cup of canned pumpkin puree
- 2 large eggs
- 2 tbsp maple syrup or honey
- 1 tsp ground cinnamon
- 1/2 tsp ground ginger
- 1/4 tsp ground nutmeg
- 1/4 tsp vanilla extract
- Pinch of sea salt
- Optional toppings: shredded coconut, cinnamon, or chopped nuts

Instructions

1. Preheat the oven to 350°F (175° C). Grease or line four ramekins with coconut oil or nonstick spray.
2. Mix the coconut milk, pumpkin puree, maple syrup (or honey), cinnamon, ginger, nutmeg, vanilla extract, and sea salt in a medium saucepan. Heat over medium heat, stirring until well mixed and warmed but not boiling.
3. In a separate bowl, beat together the eggs until smooth. Slowly pour the heated pumpkin mixture into the eggs while whisking regularly to prevent scrambling them.
4. When the mixture is fully blended, spoon it equally into the prepared ramekins.
5. Place the ramekins in a baking dish and fill with boiling water until it reaches halfway up the sides.
6. Bake for 25-30 minutes until the custards are firm but somewhat jiggle.
7. Remove from the oven and cool for 10-15 minutes before chilling in the refrigerator for at least 2 hours.
8. Serve chilled, with optional toppings like shredded coconut, cinnamon, or chopped nuts.

Nutrition (per serving):

Calories: 180 kcal Carbohydrates: 12g Protein: 5g Fat: 14g Fiber: 2g Sugars: 8g

Anti-Stress Green Smoothie

Prep Time: 5 minutes Cook Time: 0 minutes Servings: 2

Ingredients

- 1 cup of spinach or kale (fresh or frozen)
- 1/2 avocado
- 1 small banana
- 1/2 cup of coconut water
- 1 tbsp almond butter
- 1 tbsp chia seeds
- 1/2 tsp spirulina powder
- 1 tsp honey or maple syrup
- 1/2 cup of ice (optional, for extra chill)
- 1/2 tsp ground turmeric
- A pinch of black pepper

Instructions

1. Blend the spinach (or kale), avocado, banana, coconut water, almond butter, chia seeds, spirulina powder (if used), honey or maple syrup, turmeric, and black pepper.
2. Blend on high until completely smooth and creamy. If the smoothie is too thick, add more coconut water or ice until you get the ideal consistency.
3. Add honey or maple syrup to taste and adjust the sweetness as required.
4. Pour into glasses and serve immediately.

Nutrition (per serving):

Calories: 210 kcal Carbohydrates: 22g Protein: 5g Fat: 12g Fiber: 7g Sugars: 10g

Golden Turmeric Latte

Prep Time: 5 minutes

Cook Time: 5 minutes

Servings: 1

Ingredients

- 1 cup of unsweetened almond milk (or any plant-based milk)
- 1/2 tsp ground turmeric
- 1/4 tsp ground cinnamon
- 1/4 tsp ground ginger
- 1/2 tsp vanilla extract
- 1 tsp maple syrup or honey
- Pinch of black pepper
- 1 tsp coconut oil

Instructions

1. Blend almond milk, turmeric, cinnamon, ginger, and black pepper in a small saucepan.
2. Cook over medium heat, stirring regularly, until the mixture is heated (but not boiling).
3. Remove from the heat and mix in the vanilla extract, maple syrup (or honey), and coconut oil (if using).
4. Pour the golden turmeric latte into a cup, mix well, and serve warm.

Nutrition (per serving):

Calories: 120 kcal Carbohydrates: 10g Protein: 2g Fat: 9g Fiber: 2g Sugars: 7g

Ginger Lemon Detox Tea

Prep Time: 5 minutes

Cook Time: 5 minutes

Servings: 2

Ingredients

- 2 cups of hot water
- 1-inch piece of fresh ginger, sliced thinly
- Juice of 1/2 lemon (more if desired)
- 1 tsp honey or maple syrup (optional for sweetness)
- Pinch of cayenne pepper (optional, for added detox benefits)

Instructions

1. In a small saucepan, heat 2 cups of water until it boils.
2. Once boiling, add the fresh ginger slices and decrease the heat to a simmer. Allow it to cook for 3-5 minutes, depending on how strong you want the ginger to taste.
3. Remove from the heat and drain out the ginger slices from the tea.
4. Add the fresh lemon juice and honey (or maple syrup) to taste. Add a sprinkle of cayenne pepper if desired for an additional cleansing kick.
5. Pour into cups and serve immediately.

Nutrition (per serving):

Calories: 10 kcal Carbohydrates: 3g Protein: 0g Fat: 0g Fiber: 0g Sugars: 2g

Blueberry Almond Smoothie

Prep Time: 5 minutes

Cook Time: 0 minutes

Servings: 2

Ingredients

- 1 cup of fresh or frozen blueberries
- 1/2 banana (fresh or frozen)
- 1 tbsp almond butter
- 1/2 cup of unsweetened almond milk
- 1/2 tsp vanilla extract
- 1 tbsp chia seeds or flaxseeds
- 1 tsp honey or maple syrup
- A pinch of cinnamon (optional)
- Ice cubes (optional, for extra chill)

Instructions

1. Blend the blueberries, banana, almond butter, almond milk, vanilla extract, chia seeds (if using), honey, and cinnamon.
2. Blend on high until completely smooth and creamy. If the smoothie is too thick, add more almond milk or water for the appropriate consistency.
3. Add honey or maple syrup to taste and adjust the sweetness as required.
4. Serve immediately.

Nutrition (per serving):

Calories: 210 kcal Carbohydrates: 24g Protein: 5g Fat: 12g Fiber: 6g Sugars: 15g

Raspberry Ginger Lemonade

Prep Time: 10 minutes

Cook Time: 5 minutes

Servings: 4

Ingredients

- 1 cup of fresh or frozen raspberries
- 1-inch piece of fresh ginger, peeled and grated
- Juice of 3 large lemons
- 2 tbsp maple syrup or honey (adjust to taste)
- 4 cups of cold water
- Ice cubes (optional)
- Lemon slices and fresh mint (optional, for garnish)

Instructions

1. Mix the raspberries, grated ginger, and 1 cup of water in a small saucepan. Cook over medium heat for approximately 5 minutes, pressing the raspberries with a spoon to release the juice.
2. Strain the mixture through a fine mesh sieve into a large pitcher, pressing to extract as much liquid as possible. Discard the pulp.
3. Pour the lemon juice, maple syrup (or honey), and 3 cups of cold water into the pitcher. Stir well to mix.
4. Taste and adjust sweetness as needed by adding additional maple syrup or honey.
5. Add ice cubes to the pitcher or serve the lemonade over ice in individual glasses.
6. If preferred, garnish with lemon slices and fresh mint. Serve chilled.

Nutrition (per serving):

Calories: 40 kcal Carbohydrates: 10g Protein: 0g Fat: 0g Fiber: 2g Sugars: 8g

Avocado Mint Smoothie

Prep Time: 5 minutes

Cook Time: 0 minutes

Servings: 2

Ingredients

- 1 ripe avocado, peeled and pitted
- 1/2 cup of fresh mint leaves (more for garnish)
- 1 small banana (fresh or frozen)
- 1/2 cup of unsweetened almond milk
- 1 tbsp honey or maple syrup
- 1 tsp vanilla extract
- 1/4 tsp ground cinnamon
- Ice cubes

Instructions

1. Blend the avocado, fresh mint leaves, banana, almond milk, honey (or maple syrup), vanilla extract, and cinnamon (if using).
2. Blend on high until completely smooth and creamy. If the smoothie is too thick, add almond milk until you get the appropriate consistency.
3. Taste and adjust the sweetness, adding more honey or maple syrup as required.
4. Serve immediately.

Nutrition (per serving):

Calories: 180 kcal Carbohydrates: 20g Protein: 3g Fat: 12g Fiber: 7g Sugars: 10g

Anti-Inflammatory Matcha Latte

Prep Time: 5 minutes

Cook Time: 5 minutes

Servings: 1

Ingredients

- 1 tsp matcha powder
- 1/2 tsp ground turmeric
- 1/4 tsp ground cinnamon
- 1 cup of unsweetened almond milk
- 1 tsp honey or maple syrup
- 1/4 tsp black pepper
- 1/2 tsp vanilla extract (optional)
- Pinch of sea salt

Instructions

1. Mix the almond milk, turmeric, cinnamon, and black pepper in a small saucepan. Cook over medium heat, stirring regularly, until the milk is heated but not boiling.
2. Combine the matcha powder and hot water in a separate small bowl to make a smooth paste.
3. Once the milk mixture is heated, add the matcha paste and vanilla extract (if using) to the pan. Whisk together until completely blended.
4. Add the honey or maple syrup to taste.
5. Pour the latte into a cup, top with cinnamon or turmeric if preferred, and serve warm.

Nutrition (per serving):

Calories: 80 kcal Carbohydrates: 10g Protein: 2g Fat: 3g Fiber: 2g Sugars: 7g

Cucumber Mint Cooler

Prep Time: 5 minutes

Cook Time: 0 minutes

Servings: 2

Ingredients

- 1 medium cucumber, peeled and sliced
- 1/4 cup of fresh mint leaves
- 1 tbsp lime juice
- 1 tbsp honey or maple syrup
- 2 cups of cold water or coconut water
- Ice cubes (optional, for extra chill)
- Lime slices

Instructions

1. Add cucumber slices, fresh mint leaves, lime juice, and honey or maple syrup in a blender.
2. Add the cold water or coconut water and process until smooth.
3. Add honey or maple syrup to taste and adjust the sweetness as required.
4. Pour the mixture into glasses with ice cubes, if desired. Garnish with more mint leaves and lime slices.
5. Serve immediately and enjoy.

Nutrition (per serving):

Calories: 30 kcal Carbohydrates: 8g Protein: 1g Fat: 0g Fiber: 1g Sugars: 6g

Almond Butter Protein Shake

Prep Time: 5 minutes

Cook Time: 0 minutes

Servings: 1

Ingredients

- 1 tbsp almond butter
- 1 scoop protein powder
- 1/2 cup of unsweetened almond milk
- 1/2 banana (fresh or frozen)
- 1 tbsp chia seeds or flaxseeds
- 1/2 tsp vanilla extract
- 1/4 tsp ground cinnamon
- Ice cubes

Instructions

1. Mix the almond butter, protein powder, almond milk, banana, chia seeds (optional), vanilla extract, and cinnamon in a blender.
2. Blend on high until completely smooth and creamy. If the shake is too thick, add more almond milk or water for consistency.
3. Add ice cubes if you like a colder, thicker shake, then mix again.
4. Serve immediately.

Nutrition (per serving):

Calories: 250 kcal Carbohydrates: 22g Protein: 20g Fat: 14g Fiber: 7g Sugars: 10g

Strawberry Coconut Water Smoothie

Prep Time: 5 minutes

Cook Time: 0 minutes

Servings: 2

Ingredients

- 1 1/2 cups of fresh or frozen strawberries
- 1 cup of coconut water
- 1/2 cup of unsweetened almond milk
- 1 tbsp honey or maple syrup
- 1/2 tsp vanilla extract (optional)
- Ice cubes (optional, for extra chill)

Instructions

1. Blend the strawberries, coconut water, almond milk, honey (or maple syrup), and vanilla extract (if using).
2. Blend until smooth and creamy. If you like a colder, thicker smoothie, add more ice cubes and mix again.
3. Add honey or maple syrup to taste and adjust the sweetness as required.
4. Pour into glasses and serve immediately.

Nutrition (per serving):

Calories: 100 kcal Carbohydrates: 24g Protein: 1g Fat: 1g Fiber: 4g Sugars: 15g

Mango-Turmeric Smoothie

Prep Time: 5 minutes

Cook Time: 0 minutes

Servings: 2

Ingredients

- 1 ripe mango, peeled and chopped
- 1/2 tsp ground turmeric
- 1/2 tsp ground ginger
- 1/2 cup of coconut milk
- 1/2 cup of orange juice
- 1 tbsp honey or maple syrup
- 1/2 tsp black pepper
- Ice cubes (optional, for extra chill)

Instructions

1. Add the diced mango, turmeric, ginger, coconut milk, orange juice, and black pepper in a blender.
2. Blend until smooth and creamy. If you like a thicker smoothie, add more ice cubes and mix.
3. Add honey or maple syrup to taste and adjust for sweetness if desired.
4. Pour into glasses and serve immediately.

Nutrition (per serving):

Calories: 150 kcal Carbohydrates: 35g Protein: 2g Fat: 4g Fiber: 5g Sugars: 30g

Lavender Chamomile Herbal Iced Tea

Prep Time: 10 minutes

Chill Time: 2 hours

Servings: 4

Ingredients

- 2 chamomile tea bags
- 1 tbsp dried lavender flowers
- 4 cups of hot water
- 1–2 tbsp honey or maple syrup
- 1 tbsp fresh lemon juice (optional)
- Ice cubes
- Lemon slices (optional, for garnish)
- Fresh mint (optional, for garnish)

Instructions

1. In a heatproof pitcher or bowl, steep the chamomile tea bags and dried lavender in 4 cups of boiling water for 5-7 minutes.
2. After steeping, take the tea bags and filter away any used lavender flowers. Stir in the honey or maple syrup while the tea is still heated to help it dissolve.
3. Allow the tea to cool to room temperature before chilling for at least two hours.
4. If preferred, pour the iced tea over ice cubes and garnish with lemon slices and fresh mint.
5. Enjoy.

Nutrition (per serving):

Calories: 20 kcal Carbohydrates: 5g Protein: 0g Fat: 0g Fiber: 0g Sugars: 5g

28 DAYS MEAL PLAN

Day	Breakfast	Lunch	Dinner	Snacks
01	Avocado and Veggie Power Toast	Quinoa Veggie Buddha Bowl	Ginger Sesame Salmon	Cinnamon-Roasted Almonds
02	Blueberry Chia Pudding Delight	Roasted Chickpea Salad with Avocado Dressing	Moroccan Chickpea and Spinach Stew	Green Apple with Almond Butter
03	Coconut Quinoa Breakfast Porridge	Mediterranean Hummus Bowl	Herb-Crusted Tofu with Roasted Veggies	Spicy Hummus and Veggie Platter
04	Chia Seed Pancakes with Berries	Sweet Potato and Black Bean Tacos	Balsamic-Glazed Chicken with Greens	Coconut Energy Bites
05	Matcha Green Smoothie Bowl	Spinach and Chickpea Curry Wrap	Cauliflower Rice Stir-Fry	Dark Chocolate Almond Bark
06	Mushroom Spinach Frittata	Lentil & Beet Salad with Walnuts	Stuffed Bell Peppers with Quinoa and Veggies	Turmeric-Spiced Trail Mix
07	Sweet Potato and Kale Hash	Zucchini Noodle Bowl with Pesto	Thai Coconut Curry Soup	Chia Seed Crackers with Hummus
08	Almond Butter Banana Smoothie Bowl	Grilled Salmon and Greens Salad	Lemon & Herb Baked Chicken	Roasted Chickpeas with Herbs
09	Spinach & Goat Cheese Breakfast Wrap	Kale and Avocado Caesar Salad	Sweet Potato Shepherd's Pie	Baked Kale Chips with Sea Salt
10	Raspberry Coconut Yogurt Bowl	Miso-Glazed Tofu Bowl	Garlic-Roasted Sweet Potato & Broccoli	Cashew Energy Bars
11	Almond Flour Protein Waffles	Asian Ginger Salad Wraps	Zucchini and Eggplant Lasagna	Cucumber & Avocado Salsa
12	Sweet Potato Muffins	Broccoli and Almond Salad	Grilled Vegetable Paella	Zesty Lemon Energy Balls
13	Turmeric Scramble	Roasted Root Vegetable Bowl	Lentil & Vegetable Shepherd's Pie	Avocado-Cucumber Slices with Sea Salt
14	Ginger-Infused Greek Yogurt Parfait	Curried Cauliflower & Quinoa Bowl	Turmeric Chicken & Rice Pilaf	Sweet Potato Chips with Guacamole
15	Cinnamon Apple Oatmeal Bake	Spinach & Chickpea Curry Wrap	Roasted Cauliflower Steaks with Tahini Sauce	Almond Butter & Date Stuffed Apples
16	Green Veggie Omelet	Herb-Roasted Root Vegetable Bowl	Sweet Potato and Black Bean Enchiladas	Spiced Pumpkin Seed Clusters
17	Avocado & Berry Toast Duo	Detox Veggie Stir-Fry	Garlic-Roasted Sweet Potato & Broccoli	Roasted Pears with Walnuts

18	Coconut Quinoa Breakfast Porridge	Broccoli and Almond Salad	Grilled Lemon Chicken Salad	Carrot & Ginger Dip with Veggies
19	Raspberry Coconut Yogurt Bowl	Zucchini Noodle Bowl with Pesto	Herb-Crusted Tofu with Roasted Veggies	Coconut Yogurt & Berry Dip
20	Sweet Potato and Kale Hash	Lentil & Beet Salad with Walnuts	Thai Coconut Curry Soup	Dark Chocolate Almond Bark
21	Almond Flour Banana Bread	Mediterranean Hummus Bowl	Grilled Vegetable Paella	Cucumber Mint Cooler
22	Blueberry Chia Pudding Delight	Sweet Potato and Black Bean Tacos	Zucchini and Eggplant Lasagna	Lavender Chamomile Herbal Iced Tea
23	Matcha Green Smoothie Bowl	Kale and Avocado Caesar Salad	Lemon & Herb Baked Chicken	Turmeric-Spiced Trail Mix
24	Green Veggie Omelet	Spinach & Chickpea Curry Wrap	Garlic-Roasted Sweet Potato & Broccoli	Coconut Energy Bites
25	Raspberry Coconut Yogurt Bowl	Herb-Roasted Root Vegetable Bowl	Sweet Potato Shepherd's Pie	Choco-Coconut Energy Balls
26	Sweet Potato and Kale Hash	Broccoli and Almond Salad	Stuffed Bell Peppers with Quinoa and Veggies	Zesty Lemon Energy Balls
27	Cinnamon Apple Oatmeal Bake	Zucchini Noodle Bowl with Pesto	Turmeric Chicken & Rice Pilaf	Coconut Yogurt & Berry Dip
28	Avocado & Berry Toast Duo	Mediterranean Hummus Bowl	Ginger Sesame Salmon	Dark Chocolate Almond Bark

www.ingramcontent.com/pod-product-compliance
Lightning Source LLC
Chambersburg PA
CBHW081219260726
48653CB00010BB/3701